AMERICAN PUBLIC H

MW00835220

STANDARDS FOR HEALTH *in* SERVICES CORRECTIONAL INSTITUTIONS

Developed by:
APHA TASK FORCE ON CORRECTIONAL HEALTH CARE STANDARDS

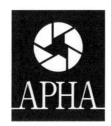

American Public Health Association
800 I Street, NW
Washington, DC 20001
www.apha.org

Georges C. Benjamin, MD, FACP, Executive Director
Mary C. White, PhD, MPH, APHA Publications Board Liaison

Printed and bound in the United States of America
Typesetting: Susan Westrate
Cover Design: Joseph R. Loehle
Set in: Melior and Eurostile
Printing and Binding: United Book Press

ISBN: 0-87553-029-X

5 M 3/03

NOTE: Any discussion of medical or legal issues in this publication is being provided for informational purposes only. Nothing in this publication is intended to constitute medical or legal advice, and it should not be construed as such. This book is not intended to be and should not be used as a substitute for specific medical or legal advice, since medical and legal opinions may only be given in response to inquiries regarding specific factual situations. If medical or legal advice is desired by the reader of this book, a medical doctor or attorney should be consulted.

The use of trade names and commercial sources in this book does not imply endorsement by either the APHA or the editorial board of this volume.

Table of Contents ———

APHA MISSION STATEMENT

The American Public Health Association is an association of individuals and organizations working to improve the public's health. It promotes the scientific and professional foundation of public health practice and policy, advocates the conditions for a healthy global society, emphasizes prevention, and enhances the ability of members to promote and protect environmental and community health.

Task Force _____

APHA *Standards for Health Services in Correctional Institutions*, 3rd Edition Task Force

Maddy deLone, MS, JD, Chair
Ms. deLone, Chair of the Task Force, is currently an attorney at the Prisoners' Rights Project of the Legal Aid Society of New York. She coordinated the development of Minimum Standards for Correctional Facilities in New York City, in her capacity as Deputy Director for the New York City Board of Correction. She has also worked to provide health services to children in detention and adult prisoners in jails in New York and has served as a correctional health expert in federal litigation involving jails.

Michael D. Cohen, MD, FAAP
Dr. Cohen, a fellow of the American Academy of Pediatrics and certified by the American Board of Pediatrics, was Chief Physician at the Adolescent Reception and Detention Center in New York City in 1985-86. Since 1994, he has been the Medical Director for the New York State Office of Children and Family Services, the state agency responsible for juvenile justice programs. In this capacity he has been responsible for the health program development, implementation, monitoring, and quality assurance for 32 state operated residential delinquency programs.

Robert Cohen, MD
Dr. Cohen served as the director of the Montefiore Rikers Island Health Services program from 1981-1986, a program which provided medical and mental health services in most of the New York City jails. He is currently appointed by the federal courts in Connecticut, New York State, and Ohio to review and monitor health care services in jails and prisons. He has reviewed the medical care provided to people in jails and prisons in many states and has published articles in the area of prison and jail health.

Ward Duel, RS, MPH

A registered sanitarian, Mr. Duel is an environmental expert and compliance consultant on the health risks associated with overcrowding and the impact of environmental conditions on inmates in correctional institutions in 44 states and the District of Columbia. In addition to appearing as an expert witness in prisoner law suits involving environmental conditions and overcrowding, he has been a Court-appointed monitor in jurisdictions including Hawaii, Missouri, Connecticut, Wisconsin, West Virginia, and Florida.

Linda Frank, PhD, MSN, ACRN, CS

Dr. Frank is an Assistant Professor, University of Pittsburgh, Graduate School of Public Health, Department of Infectious Disease. She has been the director of the HRSA-funded Pennsylvania/Mid Atlantic AIDS education and Training Center since 1988. She has been involved in prison education, training, and consultation to state correctional facilities and jails regarding the education of health care providers, peer education, and correctional education policy development to improve the quality of care since 1990. She has been the chair of the Jail and Prison Health Committee of APHA from 1996 to present.

Lambert King, MD, PhD

Dr. King's experience in prison health includes serving as a medical director and clinician at the Cermak Health Service at Cook County Jail and as the Director of the Montefiore Rikers Island Health Services. He also served from 1980–1985 as Special Master appointed by the U.S. District Court to implement a comprehensive health services system at the Menard Correctional Facility, a maximum security prison in Illinois. He has worked as an expert and monitor in numerous other prison and jail health cases and has published in the area of prison health.

Michael Puisis, DO

Dr. Puisis was the state-wide medical director of the New Mexico prison system for Correctional Medical Service. Prior to this he worked as a physician and later as Medical Director of Cermak from 1985 to 1996. He has served as a consultant to the Department of Justice on jail and prison litigation. He has also edited a textbook on correctional health care for Mosby.

Ronald Shansky, MD, MPH

Dr. Shansky served as Medical Director of the Illinois Department of Corrections from 1982-1993. He has reviewed prison and jail health services across the country as a consultant, a court appointed expert or monitor, and as an expert in litigation. Appointed by a federal district court, he served as the Receiver in a lawsuit regarding medical care in the District of Columbia jail from 1995-2000. Dr. Shansky has written and spoken extensively in the area of prison health. He is currently a consultant in correctional health.

Nancy E. Stoller, PhD

Dr. Stoller is Professor of Community Studies at the University of California, Santa Cruz. A specialist on the health of incarcerated women, she has published numerous articles and research monographs concerning the impact of the social organization of jails and prisons on access to medical care. In addition to her research, she has served as an expert witness and as a scientific consultant to non-profits, health departments, and legislators who are working to improve prisoners' quality of life.

Kim Thorburn, MD, FACP, MPH

Dr. Thorburn was a prison and jail doctor for 17 years. She provided clinical and administrative services in the California jail and prison systems and as the health care division administrator of the Hawaii Department of Public Safety. As a Kellogg National Fellow, she studied the application of health facility licensure regulations to correctional health facilities. She has inspected prisons in various capacities in the United States, El Salvador, Zimbabwe, Israel, and South Africa, and has published extensively in the field.

Corey Weinstein, MD, CCHP

Dr. Weinstein is a founder and coordinator of California Prisons Focus, a human rights and advocacy organization working with and for prisoners in California's control units since 1990. For the past 25 years, Dr. Weinstein has worked as a forensic medical expert for prisoners in class action and individual law suits in California, and he is a Certified Correctional Health Care Provider. Recently, he served as Medical Consultant for Legal Services for Prisoners with Children on the compliance team for a California case covering medical services for women prisoners in California. Dr. Weinstein coordinated the "AIDS 1995 Update" for the APHA *Standards for Health Services in Correctional Institutions*.

Contributors
and Reviewers

Amanda Anholdt, JD

Richard Belitsky, MD

Janice E. Cohen, MD

Henry Dlucacz, JD, MSW

Barbara H. Guest, MSW, MPH

Christine Johnson, RN, MPH, MS, NP

Terry Kupers, MD

Peter Kwasnik, RS, MS

Purnima Murlimanghnani, MPH

H. Whitney Payne, Jr., DDS, MPH

Ken Thompson, MD

Charles D. (Chuck) Treser, MPH

John C. Whitener, OD, MPH

Siu G. Wong, OD, MPH

Improving Palliative Care Practice in Jails and Prisons project, funded by Health Resources and Services Administration, HIV/AIDS Bureau

Preface

The publication of the Third Edition of APHA's Standards for Health Services in Correctional Institutions provides us with a moment for celebration and reflection. The American Public Health Association is proud of its quarter century association with the movement to provide access to decent medical care for the millions incarcerated in America's prisons. Against great odds, we have been more successful in improving access for this despised population than for the country at large. The credit for this effort is shared by many who have marched together under the banner and the principles of public health.

The American Public Health Association has served in the leadership of the movement to establish and protect the rights and the health of prisoners. Although there are five times as many men and women locked up today as there were when work began on the First Edition of the Standards, the effort to assure health care for prisoners has achieved successful sophisticated models of compassionate community oriented primary care within institutions dedicated to discipline and punishment.

The American Public Health Association is immensely proud of the work of the past and current editors who have defined, in their research, their practice, their politics, and their lives, the principles, the policies, and even the procedures to assure that prisoners can and do receive quality health care services.

This, of course, is a struggle which is far from over. In the continuing record of these fierce, uncompromising, yet necessary and practical standards, I believe that we are on the right track.

Quentin D. Young, MD, Past President
American Public Health Association

Introduction

We are pleased to present the Third Edition of the American Public Health Association's *Standards for Health Services in Correctional Institutions*. The "Standards" were first published in 1976. Not coincidentally, in 1976 the United States Supreme Court ruled that "deliberate indifference to the serious medical needs of prisoners constitutes the unnecessary and wanton infliction of pain . . . proscribed by the Eighth Amendment. This is true whether the indifference is manifested by prison doctors in their response to the prisoner's needs or by prison guards in intentionally denying or delaying access to medical care or intentionally interfering with treatment once prescribed." The APHA Standards were the first set of professional standards developed to assure appropriate medical care was provided to prisoners in jails and prisons.

The revised edition was published in 1986. During the intervening decade substantial progress had been made. Successive and successful litigation in state and federal jurisdictions established the constitutional requirements for prison health care. Simultaneously, and derivative from these judicial victories, successful models for the provision of medical care to prisoners were established in several jurisdictions. These programs demonstrated that decent medical care could be provided to prisoners by competent and caring practitioners given sufficient resources, dedicated leadership, and the threat of civil contempt. Under the editorship of Nancy Dubler, L.L.B., the second edition of the "Standards" defined the scope of services that were necessary to provide adequate care, basing the standards upon principles of public health and constitutional standards developed through litigation.

The second edition of the "Standards" has been extraordinarily influential in this field. It has been a popular and widely distributed APHA publication, and has been cited as the standard for jail and prison health services in state and federal court decisions which have mandated that appropriate medical care be provided to prisoners.

Why a third revision of the Standards? What has changed, what was wrong, what was missing from our previous efforts? The past fifteen years have seen a tripling of the prison population in this country. Massive outbreaks of tuberculosis, AIDS, and violence have transformed the provision of prison health in ways that must be engaged by a new set of standards. Prisons have become larger, more violent and more crowded. New forms of maximum-security prisons and punitive segregation encourage routine violence against prisoners and subject them to new and terrible forms of social isolation and psychological torture. Increasing numbers of children and adolescents are being incarcerated in more and more punitive settings.

Rehabilitation is not in the lexicon of most prison and jail administrators. Small but significant programs, such as the Pell grants, which enabled prisoners to earn college credits and degrees during their incarceration have been deliberately shut down by Congress. New and destructive laws, particularly the Prison Litigation Reform Act, have deliberately chilled the movement to litigate on behalf of prisoners' health care needs, while shutting down existing consent decrees and Court ordered oversight.

In this new environment of weakened legal support, the third edition of the Standards must be strengthened by support from the public health and medical literature to maintain the gains of the past two decades.

The Third Edition of the APHA *Standards for Health Services in Correctional Institutions* has been developed with the full realization that our job is far from over, and that providing a model of compassionate and quality health care is still critically needed in the United States. The Third Edition sets standards of health care that are respectful of prisoner patients and require prison- and jail-based health care workers to view themselves as independent health care workers first and foremost. When health care professionals identify too strongly with the security staff in the institution, they become entangled in a conflict of identity that injures them, their prisoner patients, and the institution.

These standards are based on fundamental public health principles: healthy communities, universal access, human rights, and the legal and ethical principles supporting this humane structure.

We believe the task we have set is extremely difficult but can be accomplished. We have made a number of significant changes in this edition of the Standards with the goal of getting us there. We have expanded our mental health sections substantially to begin to address the extremely complex issues faced by mentally ill prisoners and mental health professionals working in prisons and jails. We have expanded our children and adolescents section to address the needs of the increasing number of young people who are behind bars. We join with others who have called for separation of incarcerated youth and adults. We have expanded and added sections on the palliative care of prisoners with terminal illnesses which specifically address the inappropriateness of prison as a place to die, and challenge practitioners to successfully alleviate pain and suffering in an environment which is often hostile to the relief of pain.

The Third Edition addresses in detail issues of sexuality and gender in prison. It addresses the treatment of people held in isolation. We also incorporate principles set forth in international treaties that specifically address the use of torture and the provision of health care in jails and prisons. We strongly believe that these international guidelines, and possible sanctions, are of real importance to prisoners in the United States.

Some of these standards will be hard to meet, especially for small rural jails. We encourage public health systems to provide support to these small facilities to ensure that the services required by these standards are available to prisoners whether inside the jail or by formal arrangements with local government, community hospitals and clinics or individual providers.

We thank the APHA publications staff and board, the various APHA section members and other colleagues who gave their time to assist us with this effort. We also thank our families who generously gave us the time to spend on this project.

We hope these standards which describe the public health requirements of care for incarcerated persons will assist local providers in advocating and achieving appropriate conditions of confinement.

Chapter I ———————————————————————————

Organizing Principles of Care ———————————————

I.A HEALTHY COMMUNITIES

Principle: Because jails and prisons are part of the community at large, it is the responsibility of the correctional health administration to ensure that correctional facilities operate to improve the public's health.

Public Health Rationale: Correctional health services should provide public health programs for the prisoner population as well as clinical services. These services should meet relevant public health goals and objectives. The correctional health administration should also act as a liaison with local health jurisdictions (jails) or state health departments (state prison systems) to protect and promote the health of the prisoner population as well as the population of the outside community.

Satisfactory Compliance:
1. Correctional health services must have the capacity to address individual clinical needs, carry out population-wide functions, and develop and implement public health programs.
2. Public health programs in correctional facilities must have links with the appropriate public health agencies and collaborate with nonprofits and other social service agencies to ensure that the incarcerated populations' health needs are met.
3. Correctional health information systems must include preventive health maintenance schedules, surveillance data, and relevant registries, including access to adult vaccines.
4. Health promotion programs must be developed and implemented according to the needs of the prisoner population.
5. Correctional services and programs must be included in public health initiatives such as healthy community collaborations.

Cross References
Transfer and Discharge, III.H

Mental Health, V
Communicable Diseases, VI.A
Wellness Promotion and Health Education, IX

References

Glaser JB, Greifinger RB. Correctional health care: A public health opportunity. *Ann Intern Med.* 1993;118(2):139-45.

Goldkuhle U. Professional education for correctional nurses: a community-based partnership model. *J Psychosoc Nurs Ment Health Serv.* 1999;37:38-44.

Leh SK. HIV infection in U.S. correctional systems: its effect on the community. *Journal of Community Health Nursing.* 1999;16:53-63.

May J, Lambert N. Preventive health issues for individuals in jails and prisons. *Correctional Med.* 1998;259-274.

Puisis M. Update on public health in correctional facilities. *West J Med.* 1998;169:374.

Reeder D, Meldman L. Conceptualizing psychosocial nursing in the jail setting. *J Psychosoc Nurs Ment Health Serv.* 1991;29:40-4.

Skolnick AA. Correctional and community health care collaborations. JAMA. January 1998; 279(2):98-99.

U.S. Department of Health and Human Services. *Healthy People 2010.* Washington, DC: U.S. Department of Health and Human Services; 2000.

I.B   ACCESS TO CARE

Principle: Incarcerated persons have a right to health care that is quantifiable and, therefore, readily assessed at the appropriate level of care and in a timely fashion. Medical care must meet the professional standards of the community and be performed by appropriately trained and credentialed providers who are properly supervised and who use clinical protocols.

Public Health Rationale: Since jail and prison settings do not permit prisoners to spontaneously communicate their health care needs to prison staff, formal and active communication channels must be established. The urgency of any medical or mental health care problem must be determined immediately in order to provide appropriate care, avoid the spread of disease, and prevent morbidity and mortality.

Health care must be as accessed as directly as possible. The prisoner, health care staff, custodial staff, civilian staff, or other prisoners must be able to assist in the identification of a prisoner's need for care. Procedures must be developed that minimize staff discretion and minimize the ability of medical paraprofessionals or correctional officers to interfere with access to appropriate levels of care. Any triage function will only be performed by (or appropriately referred to) trained and licensed health professionals.

Prisoners in locked-down and isolated or restricted living areas (e.g., disciplinary segregation or protective custody) are most likely to experience difficulty gaining access to medical care. Systems must be in place to eliminate the barriers isolation poses to timely and appropriate health care services. And, to stem the tide of infectious disease, emergent non-discriminatory care must be available to those with HIV and other infectious diseases.

Satisfactory Compliance:

1. Upon arrival at the jail or prison, prisoners must be informed how to request medical and mental health attention. Prisoners' health care requests must be collected and reviewed daily by medical staff with triage capability and there must be a capacity for sick call at least 5 days a week. On the days without sick call, there must be the capability to handle emergencies and urgent care requests.

2. A physician should be on call at all times to answer questions regarding medical complaints.

3. Prisoners should have direct access to health care and it should not be impeded. Every health care request, other than emergency requests, must be reviewed by health care providers daily. Emergency requests should be reviewed immediately. Patients requesting a medical assessment should be triaged and seen by an independent licensed practitioner within 24 hours of the request. Medical assessments should include the gathering of subjective and objective information and an assessment and a plan based on the information gathered should be outlined in the prisoner's health record. If the prisoner is seen by a mid-level provider and continues to request examination by a physician, an examination should take place within a week.

4. Prisoners must be able to submit daily requests for medical, mental health, and dental care to health care staff whether the request is made in writing or verbally or whether the request is made by the prisoner or through other prisoners, correctional staff, cellmates, family members, or other workers in the facility. Even requests that do not arrive in the standard format must be reviewed and addressed. Prisoners with special communication needs, language barriers, mental deficits, or emotional difficulty must be identified and provided with appropriate means in which secure access to care.

5. If work is mandated, and the prisoner claims to be incapable of reporting for the assigned task due to a health issue, a face-to-face review by an independent licensed health care provider must be conducted prior to releasing that prisoner from work.

6. Prisoners may not be punished for requesting health care. Refusal of health care for a prior incident is not a valid reason to deny access to subsequent care. Prisoner-patients who perceive their health complaint as urgent must have access to care.

7. Disincentives will not be used that unduly discourage prisoners from seeking care including: copayments, sick call scheduled at unusual hours, or waiting areas that are located out-of-doors or in dangerous areas. Copayment for medical service is a tool often used in the penal system to decrease requests for medical services. Rather than raise financial barriers that make prisoners with limited funds choose between health care and subsistence items such as cleaning supplies and postage, it is more appropriate to relieve clinics of administrative functions and nonmedical referrals. Therefore, copayment requirements are considered a barrier to health care and are punitive.

8. Prisoners who complain of or display acute or emergency health problems must be referred to medical staff immediately—no matter what time of the

day or night. Prisoners with emergency situations should be evaluated onsite by a qualified licensed provider or at a community medical facility.

9. Prisoner-patients who the health care staff feels are at risk for a possible emergency must be identified and housed in an accessible area.

10. Correctional staff with emergency skills must be able to enter any living area within 60 seconds to evacuate or treat prisoners in emergency situations.

11. All prisoners who are confined to quarters or segregated must be visited by health care providers at least once a day to identify ill prisoners. A physician should make weekly rounds in all segregated areas. Health care providers must make daily log reports that include health complaints, findings and assessment, adequacy of oral intake, and a visual assessment of the prisoners' general health and welfare.

12. Unless there is a serious risk of physical harm, a segregated prisoner must be permitted to go to medical areas outside his or her housing area for assessment at the request of the health care provider. Prisoners housed in segregated areas must be examined in a clinic or medical treatment area if care is required.

13. All prisoners should be allowed consultation with their private physician on the jail or prison premises. Private physicians should have consulting, but not ordering privileges, and should communicate their recommendations to a jail or prison physician with the permission of the prisoner-patient.

14. Reasonable access to care includes access to proper medications, consultation with specialists, timely appointments, appropriate follow up of identified conditions, treatment programs, diagnostic evaluations, and discharge planning.

15. Each institution should have a written plan of care that describes and has the necessary agreements to ensure that the full spectrum of health, mental health, and dental health services are available to the prisoner population.

Cross References

Segregation, VII.D
Prisoner-Initiated Care, III.B
Follow-Up, III.C
Chronic Care Management, IV
Dental Health Care Services, VI.E
Mental Health Services, V
Urgent and Emergency Treatment, III.E

References

Lindquist CH, Lindquist CA. Health behind bars: utilization and evaluation of medical care among jail inmates. *J Community Health*. 1999;24:285-303.

New York City Board of Correction Minimum Health Care Standards.

Paris J. Sick call as medical triage. In: Puisis, M. ed. *Correctional Medicine*. St. Louis, Mo: Mosby Publishers; 1998:68-69.

Pollack H, Khoshnood K, Altice F. Healthcare delivery strategies for criminal offenders. *J Health Care Finance*. 1999;26(1):63-77.

Start A. Interaction between correctional staff and health care providers in the delivery of medical care. In: Puisis, M. ed. *Correctional Medicine*. St. Louis, Mo: Mosby Publishers; 1998:26-31.

Legal References

Davis v Dorsey, 167 F3d 411 (8th Cir 1999).

Scarberry v Bowman, 16 F3d 411 (4th Cir 1993).

Tillery v Owens, 719 F Supp 1256, 1306 (WD Pa 1989), *affd.* 907 F.2d 418 (3rd Cir 1990).

Boswell v Sherburne Cty., 849 F2d 1117, 1123 (10th Cir 1988), *cert denied*, 488 US 1010 (1989).

Mitchell v Aluisi, 872 F2d 577, 581 (4th Cir 1989).

Boswell v Sherburne Cty., 849 F2 117, 1123 (10th Cir 1988).

Wellman v Faulkner, 715 F2d 267 (7th Cir 1985).

Hoptowit v Ray, 682 F2d 1237, 1252-53 (9th Cir 1982).

Coleman v Wilson, 912 F Supp 1282 (ED Cal 1995).

Madrid v Gomez, 889 F Supp 1146, 1205-1207 (ND Cal 1995).

Arnold on behalf of H.B. v Lewis, 803 F Supp 246, 253 (D Ariz 1992)

Fambro v Fulton County, 713 F Supp 1426, 1429 (ND Ga 1989).

LeMaire v Maass, 745 F Supp 623, 636 (D Or 1990), *vacated and remanded*, 12 F3d 1444 (9th Cir 1993).

Todaro v Ward, 431 F Supp 1129 (SDNY), *aff'd* 565 F2d 48 (2d Cir 1977).

I.C ETHICAL AND LEGAL ISSUES

A. Ethical Duties

Principle: The ethical obligations of health professionals practicing in the correctional setting mirror those of health care professionals in the community.

Public Health Rationale: Professional health care ethics codify practices to ensure that patient trust is not violated and a patient–provider relationship is established so that health care can be effectively delivered. Distrust of health care providers may deter prisoner-patients from seeking health care.

Satisfactory Compliance:
1. Health care providers are the sole dispensers of medical decisions and should not be impeded by security staff or correctional administrators.
2. Clinical decisions should be guided by the best interest of the patient and should also adhere to the medical principle to first do no harm.
3. Correctional health providers' clinical skills should not be applied to nonclinical situations such as strip and cavity searches, forced transfers, health certification for punishment, or evidence gathering.
4. Health care staff are obliged to reveal medical evidence of staff brutality, including mental and physical abuse, to the appropriate authorities.
5. Health care staff should not participate in any aspect of an execution.

B. Legal Duties

Principle: The legal obligations of health care providers practicing in correctional institutions are the same as those of health care professionals who work in the community; however, health care providers within jails and prisons have an additional obligation to adhere to local, state, and federal laws that govern the provision of services to prisoners as well as the Constitution, which states that the health system cannot be deliberately indifferent to prisoners' serious medical needs.

Public Health Rationale: Health care providers in the correctional system are obliged to provide prisoners with a level of care that meets legal standards. While this standard of care is not always sufficient to meet community standards of good public health care, deviation below a legally required standard is negligent and unconstitutional.

Satisfactory Compliance:

1. Quality improvement programs must be in place to ensure that the serious health care needs of prisoners are being met.
2. The health service administration must be aware of local, state, and federal obligations regarding prison health care and must ensure that each correctional institution's health care program meets legal mandates.
3. There should be a program to educate new staff members about legal mandates for health care and to provide periodic updates for all other staff.
4. Prisoners should have access to the materials and the means to initiate legal challenges regarding medical services that they believe are unlawful under constitutional or negligence standards.

C.   Consent and Refusal

Principle: Community standards for consent and refusal of health care and treatment also apply to prisoner populations.

Public Health Rationale: Contemporary standards of health care delivery emphasize the importance of patient autonomy in health care decisions except when the public's health is threatened. These standards apply to prisoner populations as well.

Satisfactory Compliance:

1. A policy should be in place that requires voluntary informed consent prior to diagnosis and treatment. Prisoner-patients should be informed of the available health care options.
2. Consent should be witnessed by health care staff and documented in the health record prior to performing invasive procedures.
3. Prior consent may not be necessary for treatment in life-threatening or serious emergencies when time is of the essence or the prisoner is unable to give consent.
4. A policy should be in place that protects the right to refuse care. This policy should include procedures for situations in which refusal of care may present a threat to the prison population (e.g., medical isolation after refusal of tuberculosis screening).
5. Refusal of care should be witnessed by health care staff and documented in the prisoner's health record.
6. Care should be taken to ensure that refusal of care is not the result of a miscommunication or misunderstanding. Refusal of care for life-threatening conditions should be reviewed by the institution's principal medical authority. There should also be measures to involve other trusted individuals (e.g., clergy, family members) to communicate with prisoner-patients after refusal of significant care.

D.   Confidentiality

Principle: Prisoner-patients should be provided the same privacy of health care information as patients in the community.

Public Health Rationale: It is essential that prisoner-patients understand that health information is confidential.

Satisfactory Compliance:

1. A policy should be in place that protects the privacy of prisoners' health information and should include procedures for sharing health information with the correctional institution's administration when there is a threat to the well-being of the prison population.
2. When a secondary health request (e.g., special diet, special housing) is communicated to the correctional staff, the communication should not include confidential health information such as diagnoses.
3. Individual health records should be kept confidential and maintained separately from other prisoner files. Health records should not include criminal or institutional records.

E.   Prisoner Research

Principle: Since prisoners' status may subject them to potential research abuse, prisoners should only participate in biomedical research when they are treated as a protected class in accordance with federal regulations and community standards. Nevertheless, prisoners should have access to the same medical treatment as the community, including experimental treatments, as long as protections are in place.

Public Health Rationale: Biomedical research is essential to the advancement of health sciences and clinical care. But since prisoner populations have historically been exploited in the name of research, there must be protections in place to ensure that this vulnerable population benefits from research, while being protected from potential abuses. Prisoner populations have unique epidemiological features and clinical needs that can be documented through appropriate biomedical research. If the community's standard of care includes experimental treatments, prisoners should be entitled to the same potential benefits of these treatments, as long as protections are in place.

Satisfactory Compliance:

1. Prisoners should be able to participate in biomedical research, including clinical trials, provided the prisoners are given protected class status and provided that the research is also conducted on non-incarcerated populations.
2. Individual prisoner participation in biomedical research requires freely-given, written informed consent.
3. There should be no special incentive for a prisoner to participate in biomedical research.
4. All biomedical research that is available to prisoners should be authorized by an accepted institutional review board that complies with federal regulations.
5. All jail and prison health services should institute a policy regarding prisoner participation in biomedical research.

6. Under no circumstances should prisoners be permitted to participate in Phase I studies (as defined by federal regulations).

Cross References

Health Care Facilities, II.E
Staffing and Organization of Health Services, II.C

References

American Public Health Association. Policy Statement 8611, Abolition of Death Penalty. Washington, DC: APHA. 1986.

American Public Health Association. Policy Statement 2001-25, Participation of Health Professionals in Capital Punishment. Washington, DC: APHA. 2001

Anno BJ, Spencer C. Medical ethics and correctional health care. In: Puisis M, ed. *Correctional Medicine*. St. Louis, Mo: Mosby Publishers; 1998:32-39.

Dubler NN, Sidel VW. On research on HIV infection and AIDS in correctional institutions. *Milbank Q.* 1989;67:171-207.

Gostin L, Curran WJ. AIDS screening, confidentiality, and the duty to warn. *Am J Public Health.* 1987;77:361-365.

Holleran C. Ethics in prison health care. *Int Nurs Rev. 1983;30:138-40.*

Metzner JL. An introduction to correctional psychiatry: Part III. *J Am Acad Psychiatry Law.*1998;26:107-115.

Olivero JM, Roberts JB. Jail suicide and legal redress. *Suicide Life Threat Behav.* 1990;20: 138-147.

Pellegrino ED. Societal duty and moral complicity: the physician's dilemma of divided loyalty. *Int J Law Psychiatry.* 1993;16:371-391.

Smith CE. Prison psychiatry and professional responsibility. *J Forensic Sci.* 1987;32:717-724.

Thorburn KM. Nonclinical use of medical skills: beneficence lost? *Hawaii Med J.* 1995;54: 497-498.

Legal References

Legal Duties

Estelle v Gamble, 429 US 97, 104 (1976).
Fernandez v United States, 941 F2d 1488, 1493 (11th Cir 1991).
Tillery v Owens, 719 F Supp 1256, 1305 (WD Pa 1989), *aff'd* 907 F2d 418 (3rd Cir 1990).
Langley v Coughlin, 888 F2d 252, 254 (2nd Ci. 1989).
United States v DeCologero, 821 F2d 39, 43 (1st Cir 1987).
Hoptowit v Ray, 682 F2d 1237, 1246 (9th Cir 1982).
Newman v Alabama, 559 F2d 283, 291 (5th Cir), *cert. denied,* 438 US 915 (1978).

Consent and Refusal

White v Napolean, 897 F2d 103, 113 (3rd Cir 1990).
Lojuk v Quanot, 706 F2d 1456 (7th Ci. 1983).
Greer v DeRobertis, 668 F Supp 1370 (ND Ill 1983).
Kelsey v Ewing, 652 F2d 4 (8th Cir 1981).
Runnels v Rosendale, 499 F2d 733, 735 (9th Cir 1974).
Knecht v Gillman, 488 F2d 1136 (8th Cir 1973).

Confidentiality

ALA v West Valley City, 26 F3d 989, 990 (10th Cir 1994).

Nolley v County of Erie, 776 F Supp 715, 729 (WD NY 1991).
Woods v White, 689 F Supp 874, 875-6 (WD Wis 1988), *aff'd,* 899 F2d 17 (7th Cir 1990).
Doe v Coughlin, 697 F Supp 1234, 1237-38 (ND NY 1988).
Doe v Meachum, 126 FRD 437, 439 (D Conn 1988).

I.D HUMAN RIGHTS

Principle: The physical and mental health of prisoners is the most critical, as well as the most vulnerable, aspect of prison life. To promote physical and mental health, prison and jail health programs must protect and promote the basic human rights of incarcerated persons. Despite incarceration, no person should be tortured or be subjected to cruel, inhuman, or degrading treatment.

Public Health Rationale: The protection and promotion of human rights are critical elements of a humane health service program. During the past decade the United States has ratified and implemented three important international human rights treaties: Convention Against Torture and Other Cruel, Inhuman or Degrading Treatment or Punishment (CAT); International Covenant on Civil and Political Rights (ICCPR); and International Convention on the Elimination of all Forms of Racial Discrimination (ICEFRD). While the US government has declared reservations to the provisions of these treaties, and has stated that they cannot be used for direct legal redress, the treaties must inform administrative procedures.

The International Covenant on Civil and Political Rights (ICCPR) states that "all persons deprived of their liberty shall be treated with humanity and with respect for the inherent dignity of the human person." (ICCPR, Article 10/1) "The penitentiary system shall comprise treatment of prisoners, the essential aim of which shall be their reformation and social rehabilitation." (ICCPR, Article 10/2) "Each State Party... undertakes the necessary steps...to adopt such legislative or other measures as may be necessary to give effect to the rights recognized in the present Covenant." (ICCPR, Article 2/2)

The Convention Against Torture and Other Cruel, Inhuman or Degrading Treatment or Punishment (CAT) defines torture and degrading treatment and mandates that every party to the Convention undertakes to prevent such acts. "...[T]orture means any act by which severe pain or suffering, whether physical or mental, is intentionally inflicted on a person for such purposes as obtaining from him or a third person information or a confession, punishing him for an act he or a third person has committed or is suspected of having committed, or intimidating or coercing him or a third person, or for any reason based on discrimination of any kind, when such pain or suffering is inflicted by or at the instigation of or with the consent or acquiescence of a public official or other person acting in an official capacity. It does not include pain or suffering arising only from, inherent in or incidental to lawful sanctions."(CAT Article 1/1) "No one shall be subjected to torture or to cruel, inhuman or degrading treatment or punishment."(ICCPR Article 7) "Each State Party shall undertake to prevent in any territory under its jurisdiction other acts of cruel, inhuman or degrading treatment or punishment which do not amount to torture as defined in article 1...."(CAT Article 16/1)

It is the responsibility of these standards to ensure that correctional health policy and procedure is in compliance with these treaties. There is one other standing United Nations document that is essential for correctional health standards. The *Standard Minimum Rules for the Treatment of Prisoners* (SMR) was first adopted by the UN in 1955 with further approval in 1957 and 1977. It specifically refers to the *International Covenant on Civil and Political Rights* (ICCPR). The *SMR* sets out not a model system, but "what is generally accepted as being good principle and practice in the treatment of prisoners and the management of institutions."

Satisfactory Compliance:

1. "The medical services of the institution shall seek to detect and shall treat any physical or mental illnesses or defects which may hamper a prisoner's rehabilitation. All necessary medical, [dental,] surgical and psychiatric services shall be provided to that end." (SMR No. 62)

2. "The medical [staff]...should daily see all sick prisoners, all who complain of illness, and any prisoner to whom his attention is specifically directed." (SMR No. 25/1)

3. Health services in penal institutions must perform a protective as well as a therapeutic function. "The medical officer shall report to the director whenever he considers that a prisoner's physical or mental health has been or will be injuriously affected by continued imprisonment or by any condition of imprisonment." (SMR No. 25/2) Further, the medical officer "...shall visit daily prisoners undergoing...punishments and advise the director if he considers the termination or alteration of the punishment necessary on grounds of physical or mental harm." (SMR No. 32/3)

4. Jail and prison health programs should institute programs to identify and eliminate torture or other forms of inhuman or degrading treatment within the facilities.

5. Training of all staff in the institution about human rights is mandated. "Each State Party shall ensure that education and information regarding the prohibition against torture are fully included in the training of law enforcement personnel, civil or military, medical personnel, public officials and other persons who may be involved in the custody, interrogation or treatment of any individual subjected to any form or arrest, detention or imprisonment." (CAT Article 10/1)

References

The Hague. *Making Standards Work: An International Handbook on Good Prison Practice, Penal Reform International.* The Hague, Holland; 1995.

United Nations. *Universal Declaration of Human Rights. United Nations General Assembly.* New York, NY: United Nations; 1948.

Convention against Torture and Other Cruel, Inhuman or Degrading Treatment or Punishment; G.A. Res. 46, UNGAOR, 39th Session, Annex, U.N. Doc. E/CN.4/1984/E 72 (1984).

International Covenant on Civil and Political Rights; G.A. Res. 2200, UNGAOR, 21st Session, U.N. Doc. A/6316 (1966).

United Nations. *Standard Minimum Rules for the Treatment of Prisoners, United Nations Congress on the Prevention of Crime and the Treatment of Offenders.* New York, NY: United Nations; 1955.

Levy MH, Reyes H, Coninx R. Overwhelming consumption in prisons: human rights and tuberculosis control. *Health Hum Rights.* 1999;4:166-191.

Metzner JL. An introduction to correctional psychiatry: Part III. *J Am Acad Psychiatry Law.* 1998;26:107-115.

Valerio Monge CJ. HIV/AIDS and human rights in prison. The Costa Rican experience. *Med Law.* 1998;17:197-210.

Wartofsky M. The prisoners' dilemma: drug testing in prisons and the violation of human rights. *Prog Clin Biol Res.* 1981;76:57-72.

Organizational
Principles ────────────────────────────

II.A INFORMATION SYSTEMS

Principle: Jail and prison health programs must have information systems in place that allow them to monitor the performance of the health program, maintain epidemiologic information, and track prisoners' access to care.

Public Health Rationale: It is difficult to provide quality health services in jails and prisons; therefore, the system must be able to evaluate itself, look at the changing health service needs of the population, and ensure that each prisoner is appropriately monitored. Because an individual prisoner's access to health care cannot be guaranteed, it is the responsibility of the health care staff to monitor and ensure that access to care is provided.

Satisfactory Compliance:
1. The components of a health care information system must include the following:
   a. The ability to report on the services delivered by the health service program. This includes, at a minimum, the monthly number of:
      (1) New admission physicals;
      (2) Sick calls;
      (3) Immunizations;
      (4) Follow-up visits;
      (5) Specialty clinic appointments made and kept;
      (6) Emergency responses;
      (7) Emergency runs to the hospital;
      (8) Hospitalizations;
      (9) Deaths;
      (10) Use of medical restraints; and
      (11) Staff available on each shift.
   b. Collection of epidemiologic information, including prevalence data on the following:
      (1) Demographics of population (including, but not limited to, age, ethnicity, and gender);

    (2) Tuberculosis data;

    (3) HIV rates;

    (4) STD rates;

    (5) Chronic hepatitis;

    (6) Cervical cytologies (Pap tests);

    (7) Vaccination rates;

    (8) Body fluid exposures;

    (9) List of reported illnesses (by year);

    (10) Prevalence of chronic diseases;

    (11) Intentional and non-intentional injuries; and

    (12) Pregnancy rates.

  c. Means of tracking necessary medical, mental health, and dental follow-up care, including:

    (1) Immunizations;

    (2) PPD test readings (for TB);

    (3) Access to specialty care;

    (4) Periodic health assessments;

    (5) Scheduled chronic care evaluations or tests; and

    (6) Follow-up care for abnormal laboratory tests.

2. All systems, including those that are computerized, must protect the confidentiality of patient health information.

Cross References

Ethical and Legal Issues, I.C

Follow-Up, III.C

Quality Improvement, II.B

II.B QUALITY IMPROVEMENT

Principle: To ensure that the institution's health care program is consistent with standards in the community, an ongoing quality improvement program that is based on an objective evaluation of data and that corrects deficiencies found by the evaluation must operate in jails and prisons.

Public Health Rationale: To maintain and upgrade professional expertise to provide medical care that is consistent with national standards of care, all jail- and prison-based health programs must develop a system to monitor and evaluate the quality and appropriateness of patient care. This system should also facilitate the resolution of problems while pursuing opportunities to improve patient care.

Satisfactory Compliance:

A. Internal Quality Improvement

1. Each jail and prison must provide for independent internal audits of health care services and programs. These audits should be performed on a regular basis and the data generated should be documented and made available to appropriate authorities. To set standards of performance for an internal audit, multi-disciplinary teams comprised of clinical, administrative, and custodial staff must be established and should

meet every 60 days. These teams must develop a written plan outlining the health program's objectives for the year. All major health services must be evaluated for an improvement in the quality of services. In addition to assessing performance against a provider's own guidelines and protocols, services should be consistent with national community standards of professional practice and clinical services. The list of services to be reviewed annually should include, but is not limited to:

a. *Health records:* completeness as well as appropriateness of care.
b. *Institutional onsite outpatient services:* sick call and emergency services to general and segregated population prisoners.
c. *Prisoner complaints:* using prisoner complaints to gauge individual and systemic improvement strategies.
d. *Infirmary care:* notes of admission and quality of care including admission and discharge notes.
e. *Offsite specialty referrals:* timeliness and appropriateness of referrals as well as the timely receipt of specialist reports and follow up of consultation recommendations by onsite primary care physicians.
f. *Medication usage:* timeliness of medication dispensing and administration as well as appropriateness of prescribing patterns.
g. *Mental health responses:* crisis intervention, use of seclusion and restraints, incidence of involuntary medications and hospitalization, reduction in symptoms and subjective distress, improvements in social and recreational/vocational functioning, effective linkage to mental health services post-release, and methods to address complaints and grievances.
h. *Dental services:* timeliness and appropriateness of dental services.
i. *Infection control program:* use of standard precautions, sterilization procedures, aseptic techniques, and reporting and tracking of public health mandated diseases consistent with Centers for Disease Control and Prevention (CDC) guidelines.
j. *Dietary services:* monitoring therapeutic diets.
k. *Chronic care:* identification, follow up care, and monitoring for individuals with chronic illnesses such as hypertension, diabetes, asthma, seizure disorders, HIV, chronic hepatitis, and tuberculosis.

2. Health care programs must develop a written plan for a comprehensive quality improvement program and for the delegation of responsibility for the various components of the program. This plan should be updated every year.
3. Every member of the health care staff should be involved in the quality improvement program.
4. When evaluating health care services, the following performance measures should be used:
   a. Accessibility;
   b. Appropriateness;
   c. Timeliness;
   d. Continuity;
   e. Effectiveness/outcome;

    f. Efficiency;

    g. Safety of the environment; and

    h. The quality of the patient-provider interaction.

5. When the quality improvement program identifies a problem, a study should be initiated to determine the cause of the problem. Once the cause of the problem is identified, strategies must be developed and implemented to reduce or eliminate the problem. Improvement strategies may include training for staff, revision of policies and procedures, changing staffing or equipment, or reassigning clinical responsibilities.

6. Once a quality problem is identified, it must be tracked to ensure improvement or resolution.

7. The objectives, scope, organization, and effectiveness of the quality improvement program must be evaluated annually and revised as needed.

B. External Audits

In addition to the internal quality improvement process, jail or prison health systems must be audited by state or local health agencies biannually. As in the Medicare program, states may delegate the review to a non-membership national accrediting organization such as the Joint Commission on Accreditation of Health Organizations (JCAHO) or the National Commission on Correctional Health Care (NCCHC).

References

Dyer M. Quality management in the correctional health care system. *Fla Nurse.* 1993;41: 1-9.

Elliott RL. Evaluating the quality of correctional mental health services: an approach to surveying a correctional mental health system. *Behav Sci Law.* 1997;15:427-438.

Metzner JL, Dubovsky SL. The role of the psychiatrist in evaluating a prison mental health system in litigation. *Bull Am Acad Psychiatry Law.* 1986;14:89-95.

Reed TJ. Evaluating correctional health care. The lessons of New York City. *Eval Program Plann.* 1985;8:217-229.

II.C   STAFFING AND ORGANIZATION OF HEALTH SERVICES

Principle: Health services in jails and prisons must be sufficiently staffed by trained, licensed, and qualified health professionals who provide health care services that meet current national standards of care for community clinical care settings. Health care staff must also be organized and directed in a way that assures continuity, quality of care, and professional accountability.

Public Health Rationale: Jails and prisons are highly complex institutions. Increasingly technologic and specialized health care services require adequate numbers and types of qualified staff as well as careful planning to achieve current national community standards for public health and personal medical care. Health care providers within jails and prisons must be deployed, trained, and organized to meet the special needs of correctional institutions and to function as effectively as health care systems in the community.

Comprehensive health services require providers with a variety of training and licensure. Even when prisoners have medical training, allowing them to provide health care services compromises patient confidentiality and can subject the prisoner-provider to unnecessary pressure from other prisoners.

***Satisfactory Compliance*:**

1. The staff and resources of prison and jail health care programs must be of sufficient size and composition to provide prisoners with adequate health care. This requires staff for direct treatment services as well as for consultation, training, administration, evaluation, and quality improvement. The absolute number of prisoners served is not the only indicator used to determine the number of health personnel required. Experience developing adequate prison and jail health services has demonstrated that institutional physician service needs will require one full-time (FTE) physician (40 hours per week) for every 200 to 750 prisoners. Whether adequate physician staffing is closer to one FTE physician/200 prisoners or one FTE physician/750 prisoners will depend upon the following variables:

   a. Population turnover rate (turnover rates of jails are usually higher than those of prisons);
   b. Requirements for drug and alcohol detoxification;
   c. Institutional trauma and emergency incidence rates that may necessitate ongoing professional staffing;
   d. Stringent work programs that result in higher rates of sick call and medical use;
   e. Women's institutions in which medical use may be higher than in male institutions;
   f. Reception centers in which complete medical examinations are performed;
   g. Additional budgetary and staffing resources to evaluate each patient during the clinical encounter when utilization rates are greater than average.

2. The institutional health care program must have adequate financial support to maintain recruitment and the retention of trained, licensed health care staff.

3. Budgetary resources to support recruitment and employment of health care staff must be on par with the cost of care for non-incarcerated populations with additional consideration given to the special needs and dynamic nature of prison and jail populations. Budgetary and staffing decisions must also take into account the additional costs associated with security and institutional constraints, including the number of independent licensed providers necessary to provide emergency coverage.

   Adequacy of staffing must also be assessed in terms of the professional staff time available to evaluate and treat individual patients. The time available for patient encounters must be sufficient to permit prisoners to communicate medical histories; for staff to perform physical and diagnostic tests and to record findings, assessments, and treatments in prisoners' health records; and to perform patient education. Health records are useful when assessing adequacy of staffing since legible, well-documented records generally correlate to an adequacy in health care provider staffing.

4. Health services programs must be sufficiently staffed to assure proper continuity and coordination of the delivery of health services. Service coverage by physician's assistants, nurses, and administrative and other personnel must be relatively stable to assure that health services are adequately planned, delivered, and monitored. Compliance issues must also be assessed by comparing turnover and retention rates of health professionals in the institution with those of community health care organizations. Use of per diem practitioners should be reserved for emergencies.

5. Clear lines of authority, responsibility, and accountability must be maintained and the health care staff's job descriptions should be updated periodically and stay consistent with the staff's qualifications, training, and licensure status. Health care programs must designate a qualified and licensed physician as the principal medical authority. The health care program's principle medical authority must be present and onsite to meet the medical and administrative responsibilities of the position.

6. Policy and procedure manuals must contain detailed, written documentation of the program's adherence to the standards described in this book. These materials must include an organizational chart outlining lines of authority and responsibility, a contract or job description that designates the principal health authority, and staff job descriptions.

7. Experience and legal decisions have documented the need for a full- or part-time medical director to direct health services in all sizable jails and prisons. The medical director should be designated as the principal medical authority and should also be responsible for coordinating services with outside health facilities and providers. In multi-institutional prison systems, a regional or state medical director is also required; however, the need for a system-wide medical director does not obviate the need for medical directors at individual facilities. Compliance must be assessed by evaluating the size and complexity of an institutional or multi-institutional health program and comparing its requirements for a medical director with similar community systems.

8. Health care staff must be licensed and/or certified in their professional discipline and qualified to practice in a community setting. Health professionals whose licenses are restricted to employment only in state institutions are not acceptable. Qualifications of all health care staff must be on file within the offices of the institutional health care program. A working schedule of all health care providers must also be available.

9. Written policies and procedures that have been approved by the supervising physician and/or medical director must include in-service education, peer review and quality improvement as well as formal delegation of authority only to qualified and licensed providers.

10. Health-trained staff (including nurses, nurse practitioners, physician assistants, and psychologists) must not be given diagnostic or therapeutic responsibilities beyond those they are trained and qualified to assume.

11. Personnel records of health care staff must include documentation of in-service training, continuing medical education and, where required, a current certification in basic or advanced life support.

12. Health care staff must be culturally competent. A staff member fluent in the dominant languages spoken by the prisoner population should be onsite at all times. Formal arrangements with language banks or translation services should be made for all other languages.
13. Only appropriately trained and licensed staff can provide health care services to prisoners. Jail and prison health programs must be adequately funded so prisoners will not be required to work as staff.
14. Notwithstanding II.D.13, properly trained prisoners may be allowed to engage in self-help groups, peer counseling, and mutual support groups that focus on health issues such as HIV prevention and chronic disease support groups. These activities are clearly different than the prohibited use of prisoners as health providers.

Legal References

Toussaint v McCarthy, 801 F2d 1080, 1111 (9th Cir), *cert. denied*, 481 US 1069 (1987).
Wellman v Faulkner, 715 F2d 269 (7th Cir 1983), *cert. denied*, 468 US 1217 (1984).
Ramos v Lamm, 369 F2d 559 (10th Cir 1980) *cert. denied* 450 US1041 (1981).
Williams v Edwards, 547 F2d 1206, 1216-18 (5th Cir 1977).
Newman v Alabama, 503 F2d 1320 (5th Cir 1972) *cert. denied* 421 US 948 (1975).
Morales Feliciano v Gonzalez, 13 F Supp 2d 151, 209 (DPR 1998).
Inmates of Occoquan v Barry, 717 F Supp 854, 867 (DDC 1989).
Langley v Coughlin, 715 F Supp 522, 540 (SD NY 1988).
Capps v Atiyeh, 559 F Supp 894, 912 (D Or 1982).
Grubbs v Bradley, 552 F Supp 1052, 1129 (MD Tenn 1982).
Lightfoot v Walker, 486 F Supp 504, 516-17 (SD Ill 1980).
Burks v Teasdale, 492 F Supp 650, 675-678 (WD Mo 1980).
Palmigiano v Garrahy, 443 F Supp 956, 974 (DRI 1977), *remanded on other grounds*, 599 F2d 17 (1st Cir 1979).
Laaman v Helgemoe, 437 F Supp 269, 312-313 (DNH 1977).
Gates v Collier, 349 F Supp 881 (ND Miss 1972), *aff'd* 501 F2d 1291 (5th Cir1974).

II.D REFERENCE LIBRARIES

Principle: Current medical, mental health, and dental reference materials must be available for health care staff to use as a reference when treating prisoner-patients.

Public Health Rationale: Since jails and prisons may isolate health care staff from medical libraries and tertiary care centers and primary health care is often provided by physician assistants, nurse practitioners, and other non-physician providers, it is important that current reference materials be available to the staff. Internet access is also essential and should be available to download the latest clinical information and patient educational materials.

Satisfactory Compliance:

1. Current health care reference material of the following types should be available in clinics that treat the following areas:
   a. Common acute and chronic problems of adults;
   b. Common emergencies;
   c. Common skin conditions;
   d. Common OB-GYN problems (in female populations);

    e. Communicable diseases;

    f. Adolescent medicine (if the facility houses juveniles);

    g. Clinical practices;

    h. Diseases endemic to the area or population;

    i. Psychiatric diagnoses and treatment;

    j. Dental care; and

    k. Public health practices, including correctional medicine texts and journals.

II.E HEALTH CARE FACILITIES

Principle: Adequate health care facilities and staff must be available to treat and care for prisoners.

Public Health Rationale: Ready access to adequate health care facilities and personnel for prompt treatment reduces secondary infections, prolonged treatment, serious disability, and possible death. Health care services must be provided in clinical areas to establish the patient-provider relationship and ensure confidentiality and provide a safe and appropriate environment for examinations, treatment, and diagnostic testing.

Satisfactory Compliance:

1. In addition to the basic sanitary facilities, services, and practices discussed elsewhere in this book, clinic, infirmary and other medical care facilities and services must comply with the following standards:

    a. Adequate medical care and support areas must include: examination, treatment, and isolation rooms; bath and toilets; nursing stations; central and general storage; medical records storage; and separate storage space for clean and soiled linens. Sinks must have foot-, knee- or wrist-operated faucets. Examination rooms must have sinks. There must be privacy in the examination rooms and in rooms where mental health staff interview and counsel patients. Health care staff must have office space to maintain files and have access to telephones, facsimile machines, copiers, and computers with appropriate software. This equipment must be in a secured area that is accessible only to health care staff. Prisoners must have access to toilets and drinking water when they are held in waiting areas.

    b. Drugs and biologicals must be kept under lock and key, inventory controlled, and stored appropriate to their chemical, physical or biological nature. Refrigeration must be provided for pharmaceuticals when necessary.

    c. Facilities must be adequately disinfected and sterilized.

    d. There must be adequate light to perform medical tasks. Pharmacies must have at least 100 foot candles of light. Examination and treatment rooms must have 50 foot candles of light and a task-lighting level of 100 foot candles. Clinic and infirmary areas must have at least 30 foot candles of light with additional task lighting available for examination.

e. When medical or dental services are provided within the facility, equipment and analytical instruments must be provided in adequate numbers for the prisoner population's routine health needs. Institutional policies must document the required frequency and protocol for calibration and certification of all such equipment and instrumentation. At a minimum, equipment shall include:

(1) Equipment for examinations including: an examination table, blood pressure equipment with various sized cuffs, otoscope, ophthalmoscope, scale, stethoscope, nebulizer, peak flow meter, pulse oximeter, and glucose meter.

(2) Equipment for basic resuscitation (e.g., oxygen, bag, mask, oral airway, suction) and equipment for advanced resuscitation (e.g., IV, medications, laryngoscope, and automatic defibrillator (where permitted by state law).

f. Health care services may not be provided in cell or housing areas, with the exception of medical rounds discussed in the segregation section of these standards. Once health care staff determine that intervention is necessary, the prisoner must be taken to a clinical area for care.

Cross References

Ethical and Legal Issues, I.C
Segregation, VII.D
Environmental Health, X

Legal References

Harris v Thigpen, 941 F2d 1495, 1509 (11 Cir 1991).
Langley v Coughlin, 888 F2d 252, 254 (2d Cir 1989).
Williams v Edwards, 547 F2d 1206, 1217-1218 (5th Cir 1977).
Tillery v Owens, 719 F Supp 1256, 1307 (WD Pa 1989), *aff'd* 907 F.2d 418 (3rd Cir 1990).
Benjamin v Fraser, 2001 WL 359488 at *32 -*35 (SD NY).
Feliciano v Gonzalez, 13 F Supp 2d 151, 161,175,209, 211 (DPR 1998).
Palmigiano v Garrahy, 639 F Supp 244, 259 (DRI 1986).
Balla v Idaho State Board of Corrections, 595 F Supp 1558 (D Idaho 1984).
Ruiz v Estelle, 503 F Supp 1265 (SD Tex 1980).
Jones v Wittenberg, 330 F Supp 707, 718 (ND Ohio 1971), *aff'd* 456 F2d 854 (6th Cir 1972)

II.F HEALTH RECORDS

Principle: An accurate and complete health record is an essential instrument for delivery of health services and must be available for every prisoner.

Public Health Rationale: The health record enables all members of the health care staff to document health encounters and events. It also enable them to communicate critical information about the prisoner in whose care they are participating. It facilitates continuity of care when prisoners are transferred to new areas and/or institutions or when they are released to the community. An adequate medical record provides all health care staff with a comprehensive understanding of a prisoner's health problems, clinical course and management plans.

Satisfactory Compliance:

1. An individual health record must be kept for each prisoner.
2. The health record must accompany each prisoner whenever he or she is transferred to another institution or treated in a specialized area.
3. The health record must be complete, current and shall accurately reflect the health status and problems of the prisoner. Entries in the health record for each clinical encounter must include at least the following information:
   a. Date and time;
   b. Type of visit (sick call, emergency, follow-up, post-restraint, medication, procedure, etc.) and chief complaint or purpose of visit as described by the patient;
   c. Subjective (S) findings which include the patient's description of the problem or symptoms, relevant past medical history, and other observations he or she may have made.
   d. Objective (O) findings which include the clinician's observations, examination of the patient and results of any tests which are immediately available;
   e. Assessment (A) of the problem, that is, the clinician's impression of the nature of the problem or diagnosis based upon the available information;
   f. Plan of care (P), which includes, additional diagnostic studies which may be needed (i.e., laboratory, radiology, EKG, etc.); treatment to manage problem; follow-up; and instructions to the patient;
   g. Signature, printed name of provider and provider's profession (i.e., PT, MD, RN, DDS, or DMD).
4. The health record must be treated as a confidential document and shall not be released to anyone who is not a member of the health care staff, or who has not been legally authorized to receive it.
5. The health record must be kept as a unit and not fragmented by the separate health departments; medical, dental and mental health entries shall be made in the same record, but may have separate sections within it.
6. Each correctional system must standardize the format of the health record in a manner that permits information to be located easily and facilitates communication between the members of the health care staff. The health record must be organized in a manner such that professional review and quality improvement audits can be easily accomplished. Health records must include at least the following components:
   a. *Problem List:* A list at the front of the chart which enumerates the patient's significant health problems, both past and present. New problems are added as identified and the date that problems are resolved is noted. It is acceptable to separate chronic or ongoing problems from acute or self-limited problems as discrete sections of the problem list.
   b. *Flow Chart:* Patients with complex medical problems which require clinical monitoring of multiple variables over time must have a flow chart at the front of the chart which displays these results in a time sequence in an easily understood format. (e.g., sequential fasting blood sugars in a diabetic patient).

    c. *Health appraisal:* This section gathers in one place the organized base-
line health information about the prisoner which is obtained at intake
and at annual health evaluations, including comprehensive health history, physical examination, laboratory studies, and initial health screening tests.

    d. *Progress notes:* Progress notes should follow the S.O.A.P. format described
above. All medical encounters should be documented in time sequence
in the single progress notes section. Separate sections for sick call, nursing, or physician notes must not be used as this interferes with continuity of care by fragmenting the sequential recording of health information.

    e. Other sections may be designated which are deemed necessary to effec-
tively organize the health record for practical use (i.e., labs, consults,
orders, consents, etc.). Separate dental and mental health sections within the health record have been found to facilitate continuity of care in
these specialized areas.

      i) subjective complaints of the patient;

      ii) objective findings of the provider;

      iii) assessment of the problem; and

      iv) plans for continuing diagnostic, therapeutic referrals and health
education activity centering on the problem.

7. Within multi-institutional prison health systems, medical records and the
procedures by which they are prepared and maintained must be standardized to insure effective communication during inter-institutional transfers.

8. All results of outside diagnostic tests and consultations must be reviewed
and noted (countersigned) by an independent licensed provider upon receipt,
the patient shall be notified of the results, a record of the notification shall
be made, and the results shall be promptly incorporated into the patient's
health record.

9. All reports, forms, flow charts, specialty consultations, and other relevant
documents must be incorporated into the health record in a timely fashion.

10. An appropriately trained and qualified member of the health care staff must
have designated responsibility for health records in each institution, including maintenance of confidentiality, security and integrity of the records;
unique identification of each record; supervision of the compilation of
records; maintenance of the organized health record format; and maintenance of a record retention program consistent with state law.

11. Health records must be available and promptly accessible to appropriate
health care staff at all times.

12. Health record entries must be legible to other health care staff. Maintenance
of legible health records must be an integral part of the health services quality improvement program.

13. Every prisoner has the right to inspect or obtain a copy of his/her own health
record. Inspection must be arranged promptly upon request by the prisoner with health care staff available to interpret record where necessary. In no
case should there be a delay of more than two weeks in providing a pris-

oner with access to his/her health record. Copies must be made for prisoner on request, at a cost which is not prohibitive. Copies must be made available at no cost to indigent prisoners.

Cross Reference

Ethical and Legal Issues, I.C
Quality Improvement, II.B

References

Brazier, Prison doctors and their involuntary patients, *Publication Law*, 1982: 282.

Legal References

Benavides v Bureau of Prisons, 995 F 2d 269 (DC Cir 1993)
Johnson-El v Schoemehl, 878 F 2d 1043, 1055 (8th Cir 1989)
Madrid v Gomez, 889 F Supp. 1146, 1203 (ND Cal 1995)
Brown v Coughlin, 758 F Supp. 876, 882 (SD NY 1991)
Inmates of Occoquan v Barry, 717 F Supp 854, 867 (D DC 1989)
Fambro v Fulton Cty, 713 F Supp 1426, 1429 (ND Ga 1989)
Balla v Idaho State Board of Corrections, 595 F Supp 1558 (D Idaho 1984)
Cody v Hillard, 599 F Supp 1025 (SD SD 1984), *aff'd in part and rev'd in part on other grounds*, 830 F 2d 912 (8th Cir 1987), *cert. denied*, 485 US 906 (1988)
Venus v Goodman, 556 F Supp 514 (WD Wisc 1983)
Capps v Atiyeh, 559 F Supp 894 (D Oregon 1982)
Dawson v Kendrick, 527 F Supp 1252 (SD WVa 1981)
Ruiz v Estelle, 503 F Supp 1265 (SD Tex 1980), *aff'd in part and rev'd in part on other grounds*, 679 F 2d 1115 (5th Cir 1982), *cert. denied*, 460 U.S. 1042 (1983)
Burks v Teasdale, 492 F Supp 650 (WD Mo 1980)
Lightfoot v Walker, 486 F Supp 504 (SD Ill 1980)
Laaman v Helgemoe, 437 F Supp 269, 313 (D NH 1977)

Continuum of
Clinical Services _____

III.A INITIAL MEDICAL SCREENING AND COMPLETE MEDICAL EXAMINATION

Principle: Prisoners must be given an initial medical assessment by an independent licensed health care provider or a nurse with training and certification in physical assessment. The initial medical screening must precede any housing assignment other than designated intake housing. A complete medical examination must be finished within 7 days of incarceration and, when possible, the initial medical screening and the medical examination should be performed at the same time.

The examination should reflect local clinical epidemiology. Depending upon the status of the prisoner, different medical conditions will be more likely. For example, serious, acute traumas that were sustained during capture or arrest are more likely to be seen during jail intake. Newly detained prisoners are more likely to be under the influence of alcohol or drugs and are at risk for drug and alcohol withdrawal. Newly sentenced prisoners entering state or federal systems are more likely to have significant diagnosed chronic diseases requiring continuing care. However, the presence of epidemiologic variation must not affect the scope of the intake evaluation.

Prisoners held for long periods of time in municipal lock-ups often have acute medical problems. Initial medical screening conducted by licensed health professionals must take place in these facilities.

The initial medical screening examination represents the prisoner's first encounter with the medical care system. The tone of this encounter should be clinical and supportive and the independence of the medical program and the confidential relationship of provider with prisoner patient must be emphasized.

Public Health Rationale: Assessment of every prisoner's health status is essential to provide for:

1. Appropriate classification and housing;
2. Detection of health problems that require attention to protect the well being of the prisoner and the institution;

3. Gathering patient health information;
4. Collecting data on infectious diseases, injuries (e.g., accidental, preventable, and others), and chronic diseases for an epidemiologic database used for program planning and liaison with the local public health authority.

Satisfactory Compliance:

1. **Initial medical screening** (also known as receiving screening):

   a. Initial medical screenings must be performed on all individuals entering custody in an area used only for medical purposes by medical staff including trained licensed practical nurses (LPNs).

   b. Small facilities without medical staff onsite should contract with a local hospital or health facility that has licensed medical personnel to conduct initial medical screenings. There must be an established protocol to assure this initial screening takes place routinely and efficiently and that it is well documented.

   c. Initial medical screenings must begin upon entry into the facility and must be completed prior to housing the prisoner among the institutional population. In institutions with multiple housing areas, an intake area must be designated for the housing of new prisoners. Prisoners should remain in this area until the initial medical screening is performed and communicable diseases are ruled out.

   d. Health information collected from initial medical screenings should assist in determining prisoners' special housing or dietary needs as well as work and activity classification. If a prisoner is ill, the initial medical screening should be used to make housing recommendations to protect the general population from the spread of disease and should allow for appropriate treatment of the patient's condition. Prisoners with disabilities should also be identified and appropriate housing and services must be provided that accommodate their disability (e.g., wheelchair accessible cells, shower chairs, toilets that can be accessed by wheel chair dependent prisoners).

   e. Initial medical screenings of prisoners should begin with an evaluation of the prisoner's current complaints and medications, history, and physical findings followed by assessment and a problem list with a plan for each problem identified. (See Section II.C on Staffing and Organization of Health Services)

   f. Appropriate follow-up must be assured for any medical problem identified in the initial screening. For example, medications must be continued without interruption. Adequate stocks of medication must be available onsite to assure there is no disruption of treatment for patients with HIV infection, hypertension, epilepsy, diabetes, or other diseases where continuity of treatment is critical.

   g. The initial medical screening and the complete medical examination should be recorded on a form and should include all of the required elements listed in this section.

   h. Medical records from other institutions should be added to prisoners' current institutional health records. Signed consent is required when requesting health information from other institutions. When health information, such as medication identification, is needed urgently, appropriate phone calls should be made (with the prisoner's permission) and the information documented in the health care record.

i. It is the institution's responsibility to maintain communication with the prisoners; therefore, personnel must be available to communicate with prisoners with language barriers (e.g., deaf, non-English speaking).

j. Initial medical screenings should provide the appropriate setting to inform the prisoner of the institution's procedures for requesting medical attention.

k. Initial medical screening of the prisoner, as with all health care, must be carried out in a clean space with visual and aural privacy to assure the accuracy and confidentiality of the information gathered. Health care should not be provided through the bars or openings in cell doors.

l. The examination area must have adequate light and should be equipped with hand washing facilities and appropriate equipment as described in the facilities section of these standards. The patient should be clothed in a garment suitable for examination. Correctional staff of the same gender should provide security when a prisoner is not dressed. To maintain confidentiality, correctional staff must maintain a distance that provides aural privacy.

2. **The initial medical screening must identify prisoners with:**
   a. Drug withdrawal or prisoners at risk of drug withdrawal. Withdrawal should be noted in the health record;
   b. Painful conditions or injuries;
   c. Medical emergencies requiring treatment;
   d. Chronic diseases requiring ongoing treatment;
   e. Mental health problems, particularly severe depression and suicidal ideation, and prisoners who require emergency or urgent psychiatric evaluation. If a potential mental health emergency is identified, there must be immediate access to an independent licensed mental health provider; and
   f. Communicable diseases.

3. **The initial medical screening must also include:**
   a. Vital signs (e.g., blood pressure, pulse, temperature, respiratory rate, and weight);
   b. Observation of exposed skin for the presence of jaundice, abscess, rash, or infestation;
   c. Examination and documentation of recent trauma;
   d. Evaluation of mental status, including level of alertness, anxiety, depression, or psychosis; and
   e. Respiratory status.

4. **The following activities *must not* be part of initial medical screening:**
   a. Body cavity searches;
   b. Forensic examination of hair and/or blood;
   c. Evaluation for suitability for restraint by stun gun weapons, noxious gases, or restraint boards; and
   d. Involuntary testing for HIV infection.

5. **Required intake laboratory and diagnostic studies:**
Most prisoners who are detained remain in jail less than 2 weeks, while most prisoners in state and federal institutions are incarcerated for an average of 2 years. Therefore, it is reasonable to differentiate the laboratory and diagnostic tests used to screen for medical problems in these populations.
   a. Laboratory tests for newly detained prisoners should include:
      (1) Rapid serologic test for syphilis with a confirmation test for false-positive test results;
      (2) PPD implantation and/or chest radiograph for tuberculosis;
      (3) Urine pregnancy test;
      (4) Chlamydia and gonorrhea urine screening for men; and
      (5) Urinalysis.
   b. Additional laboratory studies that are part of the complete physical examination:
      (1) Cervical cytology (Pap test) and cervical screening for chlamydia and gonorrhea;
      (2) Electrocardiograms for patients older than 40;
      (3) Hepatitis B antibody screening (and access to immunization for Hepatitis B);
      (4) Hepatitis C screening; and
      (5) All laboratory tests required to identify chronic diseases.
   c. An additional laboratory test for sentenced prisoners or for detained prisoners whose stay exceeds 3 months is a CBC and SMA-20 or equivalent (must include fasting blood sugar and cholesterol).
6. **The complete medical examination:**
   a. The complete medical examination is a comprehensive evaluation performed after the initial medical screening. A complete medical examination should take place as soon after admission as possible (preferably before the seventh day after admission). Additional historical information obtained at this time should include:
      (1) Medical, surgical, and family histories;
      (2) Medications (past and present use);
      (3) Prior hospitalizations, including psychiatric hospitalizations and history of tuberculosis;
      (4) Past history of sexual abuse;
      (5) Sexual orientation including high-risk sexual behavior;
      (6) Allergies and immunization status; and
      (7) Obstetrical history.
   b. If vital signs are obtained by the nursing staff, a comprehensive physical examination can be completed within 10 to 15 minutes. Prior to the examination, the patient must be provided with a gown to facilitate complete visualization of the body. All systems and organs must be examined including:
      (1) Head
      (2) Eyes (including vision screening)
      (3) Ears (including hearing screening)
      (4) Nose

(5) Mouth and throat
(6) Teeth
(7) Neck
(8) Thyroid
(9) Lymph nodes
(10) Pulses
(11) Heart
(12) Lungs
(13) Chest/breast
(14) Abdomen
(15) Hernia
(16) Genital
(17) Rectal
(18) Musculoskeletal, including range of motion of limbs
(19) Feet
(20) Neurological system
(21) For prisoners 40 and older, tonometry must be measured and a baseline electrocardiogram must be performed.

There must be particular emphasis and comment on the presence or absence of abnormalities suggested by the medical history and the examination must be well documented in the medical record and all abnormalities must be described in appropriate clinical detail.

7. **Initial mental health screening**

The initial mental health screening must be performed by a trained health professional sensitive to the mental status and possible mental illness of the prisoner. The evaluation, which must be done contemporaneously with the initial medical screening must include:

a. Mental health history including history of mental illness, mental health treatment (including medications), education, work history, social history, sexual history and orientation, and family drug and alcohol use;
b. Assessment of coping mechanisms including any indications by the prisoner of a desire for help;
c. Identification of psychosis or suicidality;
d. Evaluation of the need for referral to mental health services; and an
e. Explanation of the mental health services available, procedure for application, and referral if requested.

Mental health screenings must be documented in the prisoners' medical record.

8. **Medical classification**

After the initial medical screening and the complete medical examination are completed and the findings evaluated, certain prisoners may be medically classified and assigned to special housing areas. The following medical categories must be considered in identifying inmates who may require medical classification and possible separation for appropriate diagnosis and treatment:

a. Those with communicable diseases;

   b. The physically weak and infirmed;

   c. The mentally retarded and demented;

   d. Those requiring mental observation because of risk of suicide or severe thought disorder;

   e. The chronically ill and debilitated; and

   f. Those at extremes of the age spectrum, young or old.

9. **Assessment and plan**

For each new prisoner, a medical and mental health status assessment should be prepared and a plan for appropriate follow-up care for all abnormalities as well as necessary health maintenance should be developed. Where indicated, specialty medical housing areas will be recommended. The assessment and plan should be completed and detailed on a preprinted medical intake form, signed, and time and date of completion noted.

Prisoners diagnosed with chronic diseases will have disease specific comprehensive laboratory and diagnostic testing as part of their initial evaluation. Immunizations will be provided, based upon CDC recommendations, including Diptheria/Tetanus, Influenza, Pneumococcal, Hepatitis B, as well as Hepatitis A for all prisoners with Hepatitis C infection.

10. **Refusal of intake examination**

   a. Every prisoner has the right to refuse a medical examination; this right must be respected.

   b. Any prisoner who refuses the intake examination must be placed under daily medical observation and a plan must be developed to evaluate them for placement in an appropriate housing area.

   c. Mentally ill persons should be identified and, if necessary, legal proceedings initiated to address the problems of the patient who fits criteria for involuntary treatment.

   d. The confused, disoriented prisoner may require medical hospitalization.

   e. All prisoners who are placed in segregated housing for medical observation must be interviewed daily by a health professional, and at least every other day by a physician.

   f. Policies developed to implement items 10a-e should be implemented by the least restrictive procedures consistent with the possible risk to the prisoner and to others in the institution.

Cross References

Access to Care, I.B
Mental Health Services, V
Health Services for Women, VII.A
Children and Adolescents, VII.B

References

Cohen, RL. Intake evaluation in prisons and jails. In: *Clinical Practice in Correctional Medicine*, Puisis M, ed. St. Louis, Mo: Mosby Publishers; 1998.

Lessenger, JE. Health care in jails: a unique challenge in medical practice. *Postgrad Med.* 1982; 72: 3.

Legal References

Madrid v Gomez, 889 F Supp 1146, 1204-1205 (ND Cal 1995).
Fambro v Fulton Cty, Ga., 713 F Supp 854, 867 (ND Ga 1989).
Inmates of Occoquan v Barry, 717 F Supp 854, 867 (DDC 1989).
Tillery v Owens, 719 F Supp 1256, 1306 (WD Pa 1989), *aff'd* 907 F2d 418 (3rd Cir 1990).
Palmigiano v Garrahy, 639 F Supp 244, 259 (DRI 1986).
Cody v Hillard, 599 F Supp 1025, 1059 (DSD 1984), *aff'd in part and rev'd in part on other grounds*, 830 F2d 912 (8th Cir 1987) (en banc), *cert. denied,* 485 US 906 (1988).

III.B PRISONER-INITIATED CARE (SICK CALL)

Principle: Sick call is a system for non-emergency patient-initiated health care. If facilities use nurses to screen prisoners' medical requests, there must be a system to ensure that prisoners see mid-level practitioners or physicians when they need higher levels of care.

Public Health Rationale: Given the restricted movement in correctional settings, systems must be developed to ensure that health needs can be communicated to and evaluated by the appropriate medical staff.

Satisfactory Compliance:

1. Sick call must be an organized system conducted by a physician, or by a licensed mid-level practitioner under the daily supervision of a physician. Nurses (RNs) who conduct sick call must have documented training in physical assessment, and they must conduct sick call under written standing orders for management of common self-limited conditions. RNs must refer conditions not covered by standing orders or conditions not responsive to routine care to physicians or mid-level practitioners. Conditions are considered to be not responsive to routine care if the patient is seen twice for the same complaint with no improvement.
2. Sick call should be available at least 5 days a week.
3. Prisoners requesting care must be scheduled for sick call on the next day sick call is held after it is determined by medical staff that immediate, emergency care is not necessary.
4. Sick call must be carried out in a private area that permits confidential and linguistically and culturally appropriate communication between patient and practitioner.
5. All decisions regarding referral to medical staff must be made by health care providers.

References

Paris JE. Sick call as medical triage. In: *Clinical Practice in Correctional Medicine.* Puisis M, ed. St. Louis, Mo: Mosby Publishers; 1998.

Legal References

Fields v City of South Houston, Texas, 922 F2d 1183, 1192, n.10 (5th Cir 1991).
Hoptowit v Ray, 682 F2d 1232, 1252-3 (9th Cir 1982).
Williams v Edwards, 547 F2d 1206 (5th Cir 1977).
Tillery v Owens, 719 F Supp 1256, 1306 (WD Pa 1989), *aff'd* 907 F2d 418 (3rd Cir 1990).

Palmigiano v Garrahy, 639 F Supp 244, 259 (DRI 1986).
French v Owens, 538 F Supp 910 (SD Ind 1982), *aff'd in part, reversed in part,* 777 F2d
    1250 (7th Cir 1985).
Balla v Idaho State Board of Corrections, 595 F Supp 1558 (D Idaho 1984).
Ruiz v Estelle, 503 F Supp 1265 (SD Tex. 1980), *cert denied*, 103 S Ct 1438 (1983).
Todaro v Ward, 431 F Supp 278 (SD NY 1977).

III.C FOLLOW-UP

Principle: There must be follow-up care for every health problem identified in the initial medical screening, the complete medical examination, sick call visits, or any other health care encounter.

Public Health Rationale: The structure and operation of correctional systems (jails in particular) make ready response to the ongoing health care needs of prisoners difficult. Most jail and prison systems have been based on the sick call model, which was designed for the episodic needs of healthy young people in military service. An aging prison population with serious chronic health needs requires carefully planned follow-up services. Follow-up care is essential to the proper continuity of care within a jail or prison and when prisoners are transferred to other facilities or released.

Satisfactory Compliance:

1. Every medical interaction must generate an assessment and a plan. Every plan recorded must include some statement of follow-up care that must be carried out in a timely fashion.

2. Abnormal findings from the screening history, physical exam, laboratory results, or other source must be noted and systematically evaluated and managed by a physician or mid-level practitioner.

3. Chronically ill patients must be evaluated at regularly determined intervals. Patients with stable chronic conditions must be seen and evaluated at least quarterly by a physician or mid-level provider. Other prisoners that require quarterly medical appointments are those undergoing any ongoing treatment program, or those with a disability that prevents ordinary housing or programming.

Cross Reference

Chronic Care Management, IV

References

Puisis M, Robertson JM, Chronic disease management. In: *Clinical Practice in Correctional Medicine*. Puisis M, ed. St. Louis, Mo: Mosby Publishers; 1998:51-66.

Legal References

Hinson v Edmond, 192 F3d 1342 (11th Cir 1999).
Hemmings v Gorczyk, 134 F3d 104, 109 (2nd Cir 1998).
Creech v NGuyen, 153 F3d 719 (4th Cir 1998).
Harris v Greifinger, 172 F3d 37 (2nd Cir 1998) (Unpublished).
Miller v Schoenen, 75 3d 1305 (8th Cir 1996).

Lightfoot v Walker, 486 F Supp 504 (SD Ill 1980).
Newman v Alabama, 349 F Supp 278 (MD Ala 1978).
Todaro v Ward, 431 F Supp 1129 (SDNY 1977).
Goldsby v Carnes, 365 F Supp 395 (WD Mo 1973), *modified* 429 F Supp 370 (1970).

III.D SPECIALTY CONSULTATIVE SERVICES

Principle: Specialty consultants are needed to provide care that is not within the expertise of the institution's regular medical staff and must be available.

Public Health Rationale: Consultation with specialists for prisoners' special medical needs is critical for comprehensive health care. Communication with specialists maintains the level of care at the current national standard of community care, is an essential source of continuing education and patient-specific information, and helps integrate the correctional medical staff into the local and regional medical care community.

Satisfactory Compliance:
1. Every jail and prison health care program must have a comprehensive roster of specialty consultants who are available onsite or readily accessible outside the institution.
2. Consultants in all ordinary specialties, and those required for specific local needs, should be contracted by prior verbal and written agreement whenever possible.
3. All routine specialty service providers must have standing contracts with the facility.
4. Referral to specialty consultants to evaluate and treat problems beyond the capability of the medical staff of the institution should be ordered by the attending physician. In facilities serving children, pediatric specialists should be used to manage problems unique to childhood.
5. Facility medical staff must determine whether the need for outside consultation is an emergency, urgent, or non-urgent. Immediate referral is required in any emergency situation. Urgent referral is required for prisoners with illnesses not responding or responding poorly to present management, or who may deteriorate if left untreated, or for painful conditions uncontrolled by routine analgesia. An appointment for urgent care must be scheduled within 2 weeks of the referral, unless an earlier appointment is clinically required. Non-urgent specialty appointments should occur within 4 weeks of the referral. Routine screening tests (e.g., colonoscopy or mammography) that require outside consultation, must be scheduled within a time frame requested by the independent licensed providers. Time frames required by these provider staff must be honored.
6. Written procedures must be developed to assure timely appointments, transportation (if necessary) and follow-up. Adequate vehicles and correctional personnel must be available to transport prisoners to outside medical facilities when it is deemed necessary by the medical staff. Vehicles used to transport prisoners with disabilities must be outfitted consistent with national community standards for similar vehicles and must include safety restraint

systems. Specialty appointments should not be subject to disincentives like excessive travel time, painful restraints, missed meals, and housing changes.

7. Verbal and written consultation reports must be conveyed to the referring physician and placed in the patient's chart.

8. A consultant's recommendations must be reviewed and acted upon. Correctional and medical staff are responsible for assuring that consultant advice is received and followed. If a consultant's recommendations are not to be carried out, reasons and actions must be charted.

9. Formal guidelines should determine the approach to non-urgent problems.

10. Specialty consultation to the appropriate level of care should be required for all chronically ill prisoners with significant functional deficit who have a condition that is deteriorating. Factors often considered in determining the approach to treatment of non-urgent problems include: length of stay of the prisoner in the institution, length of time the medical condition has existed, whether it is necessary to prevent long term damage or disability, or whether the treatment tends to contribute to rehabilitation goals (including employability, physical ability, and education), and whether it relieves pain and suffering. All conditions for which failure to treat would hasten the worsening of the condition must be treated in a timely fashion. If time does not permit the completion of a therapeutic intervention or public health measure, appropriate referral must be made to a community health care setting. The approval and utilization processes should not delay care.

11. The providers of specialty services should have personnel files at the institution in which their credentials are kept up-to-date and should also include medical license, CV, board certification, and hospital privileges. In jails or prisons where a hospital provides medical staff, credentialing may be delegated to the hospital; however, board certified specialists are preferred. At a minimum, specialists must be board eligible. Their work should be reviewed annually by the principal medical authority and staff, and their relationship with the institution should be maintained or discontinued depending on the results of the annual evaluation.

Cross References

Access to Care, I.B

Distance-Based Medicine, VI.H

References

Puisis M. Chronic disease management. In: *Clinical Practice in Correctional Medicine.* Puisis M, ed. St. Louis, Mo: Mosby Publishers; 1998.

Legal References

Hunt v Uphoff, 199 F3d 1220 (10th Cir 1999).

Hemmings v Gorczyk, 134 F3d 104, 109 (2nd Cir 1998).

Waldrop v Evans, 871 F.2d 1030, 1036 (11th Cir), *rehearing denied*, 880 F2d 421 (11 Cir 1989).

Tillery v Owens, 719 F Supp 1256, 1307 (WD Pa 1989), *aff'd*, 907 F2d 418 (3rd Cir 1990).

Ancata v Prison Health Services, Inc., 769 F2d 700, 704-05 (11th Cir 1985).

Matzker v Herr is 748 F2d 1142, 1147 (7th Cir 1984), *overruled on other grounds, Salazar*
   v City of Chicago, 940 F2d 233, 240 (7th Cir 1991).
West v Keve, 571 F2d 158, 162 (3rd Cir 1978).

III.E   URGENT AND EMERGENCY TREATMENT

Principle: Emergency care and access to urgent medical treatment must be available to prisoners in a safe and timely fashion 24 hours a day. The care provided must be on par with accepted contemporary national standards for community care.

Public Health Rationale: Access to medical care outside of the sick call process is severely limited in prisons and jails; however, serious painful medical conditions as well as clinical emergencies can and do occur. Access to urgent care can prevent the development of many emergencies. A prisoner can request urgent care based upon his or her perception of need; and the request must be heeded. Correctional staff who are trained to recognize and respond to emergency situations will reduce harm to the population. A well-designed emergency care system that is integrated into the regional 911 system must exist at each correctional facility.

The clinical epidemiology of prisons and jails underlines the need to provide well-designed and adequately-staffed emergency response to a variety of medical events including life threatening trauma from penetrating wounds, poisonings, suicide attempts, uncontrolled epilepsy, and status asthmaticus as well as cardiac emergencies. Traumatic injuries and cardiac events are common for prisoners and for corrections staff.

Some medical emergencies can be prevented by public health efforts. This can be accomplished by controlling (decreasing) the level of violence within jails and prisons and by having well-designed systems to manage chronic illnesses and thereby decrease the incidence of hypertensive, asthmatic, and epileptic emergencies. Identification of prisoners with severe depression, compassionate and effective mental health treatment, and prompt emergency access to mental health professionals, including psychiatrists, can dramatically decrease the number of attempted suicides in prisons and jails.

National standards have been developed over the past ten years to assure prompt access to emergency care for non-incarcerated persons. The systems are built around networks of community hospitals, emergency transportation (ambulance) capacities including continuous hospital monitoring of critically ill patients during transport, and trauma centers of increasing capacity. Prisoners must have access to the level of care that they need and must not be limited to the care available at the jail or prison if that care is inadequate.

Satisfactory Compliance:

1. Prisoners who request to see the health care staff for an urgent or an emergency medical condition must be given access to care.
2. The request for urgent or emergency medical care must not result in discipline.
3. Health care and correctional staff will jointly develop protocols to ensure an effective and immediate response to all medical emergencies. These pro-

tocols will include a clearly identified "first responder" from the health care staff available on every tour. The "first responder" should be able to reach any critically ill prisoner within 4 minutes. Appropriate emergency equipment for handling emergencies must be available and should, at a minimum, include: bag, mask, oral airway, oxygen, suction, IV, fluids, and drugs (e.g., glucogon, epinephrine). Compliance with this requirement will be documented quarterly.

4. Medical and correctional staff will be trained and certified in CPR as well as first aid and emergency skills. Correctional staff will be required to initiate CPR immediately rather than waiting for the arrival of medical staff. Every housing and program area should be supplied with gloves, face mask, one-way oral tube, first aid kits, and spill kits. At each facility, at least one physician will be ACLS certified.

5. Protocols for the emergency management of status asthmaticus, uncontrolled hypertension, myocardial infarction, status epilepticus, hanging, drug overdose, hypogclycemic crisis as well as blunt and penetrating trauma must be developed and be consistent with national standards for community emergency care. The medical staff must be trained to follow these protocols.

6. Prisoners suffering medical emergencies that cannot be appropriately treated at the correctional facility will be transported to the closest facility with the appropriate emergency capability.

7. Liaison with local 911 emergency vehicle transport should be established and be available to prisoners as well as correctional personnel when needed. 911 vehicles should have direct access to the medical area to expedite emergency transfers to outside hospitals. In non-life threatening emergency transport situations, appropriately equipped facility vehicles may be used to transfer prisoner patients from the correctional facility to the appropriate hospital. All vehicles that transport disabled prisoners must be outfitted consistent with national community standards.

8. Automatic external defibrillators, if permitted under state law, should be available for use during cardiac emergencies.

9. Health care providers must be involved in the formulation of disaster plans in the event of fire or other natural disasters.

10. Disaster plans and evacuation plans should include quarterly drills to maintain familiarity with the plan and assure its successful implementation.

Cross Reference

Access to Care, I.B

Legal References

Sealock v Colorado, 218 F3d 1205 (10th Cir 2000).
Sherrod v Lingle, 2000 WL 1046586 (7th Cir 2000).
Green v Carlson, 581 F2d 669 (7th Cir 1978), *aff'd* 446 US 14 (1980).
Madrid v Gomez, 889 F Supp 1146, 1257. (ND Cal 1995).
Balla v Idaho State Board of Corrections, 595 F Supp 1558 (D Idaho 1984).
French v Owens, 538 F Supp 910 (SD Ind 1982).
Lightfoot v Walker, 486 F Supp 504 (SD Ill 1980).

Burks v Teasdale, 492 F Supp 650, 678 (WD Mo 1980).
Nelson v Collins, 455 F Supp 727 (D Md 1978).
Laaman v Helgemoe, 437 F Supp 269 (DNH 1977).
Palmigiano v Garrahy, 443 F Supp 956 (DRI 1977).

III.F SECONDARY CARE SERVICES (HOSPITAL AND INFIRMARY CARE)

Principle: Every jail and prison must plan and assure timely availability of a range of health services beyond those that can be provided on an ambulatory basis.

Public Health Rationale: Because prisoners are not autonomous in seeking more specialized health care, it is incumbent upon the health services staff and the corrections agency to plan for and ensure that a full continuum of quality health services will be available when needed. The nature of access to all levels of care is as important in determining the quality of care as are the specific aspects of care rendered. Services required beyond outpatient care in the correctional institution include diagnostic evaluation, observation, convalescent and rehabilitative care, medical and psychiatric hospitalization, long term care, and hospice care.

Satisfactory Compliance:

1. Each correctional health program must have a written patient care plan that defines its arrangements and procedures for the delivery of health services beyond those available on an ambulatory basis. The patient care plan should include a full continuum of health services including hospitalization for both medical and psychiatric services in facilities that are accredited by the Joint Commission on Accreditation of Healthcare Organizations (JCAHO) and licensed by applicable state and local health agencies.

2. The use of local community hospitals and more specialized tertiary care hospitals for treatment of prisoner needs must be arranged in advance to ensure timely transportation, provision for any security measures that are necessary, appropriate discharge planning, and confidential transmittal of medical information such as discharge summaries that must accompany the patient.

3. Hospital services operated by or used by correctional institution's agencies must be accredited by the JCAHO under its applicable standards and meet state and local licensure requirements for facilities serving the public.

4. Correctional institutions operating ambulatory surgery units or infirmaries, long term care, rehabilitation or observation areas, including facilities that provide pre-hospital and/or pre-surgical evaluation and care and post-hospital and/or post-operative care must be accredited by the JCAHO under its applicable standards and meet state and local licensure requirements for comparable facilities serving the public.

5. All care provided in secondary care facilities, both inside and outside the institution, must be regularly evaluated as part of the health services quality improvement program. Written records of such evaluation must be maintained.

Cross References

Access to Care, I.B

Quality Improvement, II.B

References

Braslow CA. Comment quality of care includes access to care. *J Prison Jail Health*. 1990; 9:155-157.

Brecher EM, Della Penna R. *Prescriptive Package-Health Care in Correctional Institutions*. Washington, DC: National Institute of Law Enforcement and Criminal Justice, Law Enforcement Assistance Administration, US Department of Justice; 1975.

Heyman B: The hospital secure unit. In: *Clinical Practice in Correctional Medicine*. Puisis M, ed. St. Louis, Mo: Mosby Publishers; 1998:86-98.

Weisbuch JB. The new responsibility for prison health. *J Prison Jail Health*. 1991;10:3-18.

Legal References

Hoptwit v Ray, 682 F2d 1237 (9th Cir 1982).

Jackson v State of Mississippi, 644 F.2d 1237 (5th Cir 1981).

Madrid v Gomez, 889 F Supp 1146, 1257 (ND Cal 1995).

Capps v Atiyeh, 559 F Supp 894 (D Or 1982).

French v Owens, 538 F Supp 910 (SD Ind 1982).

Ruiz v Estelle, 503 F Supp 1265 (SD Tex 1980).

Feliciano v Barcelo, 497 F Supp 14 (DPR 1979).

III.G PERIODIC HEALTH ASSESSMENT

Principle: Prisoners must have access to regularly scheduled health evaluations consistent with national community standards of care.

Public Health Rationale: Disease prevention and periodic health assessments are integral components of any public health approach to health service delivery. With restricted access to care and high levels of morbidity and need, jails and prisons must have strong programs to identify and manage health problems and promote wellness and education of patients. Periodic health assessments are part of such a program. Periodic health evaluations also provide an opportunity to intervene with patients to reduce risky behaviors (e.g., smoking cessation, low fat and cholesterol diet, anger control, and standard precautions to avoid blood and body fluid exposures).

Satisfactory Compliance:

1. Periodic health assessments of prisoners should be performed and recorded in the medical record. These periodic assessments should meet the requirements of the United States Preventive Health Services Task Force as to content and frequency. At a minimum, the periodic assessment should include:
   a. Interval health history and review of systems that may be completed by the literate patient through the format of a written questionnaire that is reviewed and followed up on by an independent licensed provider;
   b. Physical exam including weight and vital signs;
   c. Visual acuity testing;
   d. Dental exam;

e. Mantoux PPD testing if prior negative;

f. Hearing assessment;

g. Serologic test for syphilis after the first year in custody; and

h. At age 40: baseline EKG.

i. Over age 40:

    (1) Rectal exam and stool test for occult blood; and

    (2) Tonometry.

j. Immunizations (when indicated):

    (1) Flu vaccine;

    (2) Pneumococcal vaccine;

    (3) Tetanus/diphtheria immunization (TD);

    (4) Hepatitis B and C vaccines; and

    (5) Chickenpox vaccine.

k. Women:

    (1) Breast exam;

    (2) Cervical cytology (Pap test); and

    (3) Mammography when indicated.

2. Other tests as indicated including testing for endemic disease in the population.

3. Health problems suspected or identified should be evaluated and treated with appropriate follow-up care.

Cross Reference

Wellness Promotion and Health Education, IX

References

Brewer MK, Baldwin D. The relationship between self-esteem, health habits, and knowledge of BSE practice in female inmates. *Public Health Nursing.* 2000;17(1):16-24.

Spitzer WO. Canadian task force on the periodic health examination. The periodic health examination: 1984 Update. *Can Med Assoc J.* 1984;130:1278-1285

Guide to Clinical Preventive Services: Report of the U.S. Preventive Services Task Force.

Legal References

Madrid v Gomez, 889 F Supp 1146, 1257-1259 (ND Cal 1995).

III.H TRANSFER AND DISCHARGE

Principle: There must be a plan for continuity of care, whether a prisoner is transferred to another correctional system or facility or returned to the community.

Public Health Rationale: An aging population with serious chronic health care needs and a population with high prevalence of chronic and infectious disease require carefully planned systems to ensure continuity of services upon transfer to other facilities or upon release to the community.

Satisfactory Compliance:

1. Medical staff must be given timely notice of prisoners' anticipated transfer or release from the institution in order to prepare records, medications, and follow-up referrals in advance.

2. The complete health care record must accompany a prisoner who is transferred *within* a correctional system. A system must be in place to notify the medical providers in the receiving institution when prisoners are being transferred who require immediate or uninterrupted treatment for chronic or ongoing medical or mental health conditions. The complete record must be reviewed by a registered nurse, physician, or mid-level practitioner on the day of the prisoner's arrival at the receiving institution. This review must be noted in the chart.

3. When prisoners are transferred between correctional systems, a transfer summary must be forwarded to the receiving institution. At a minimum, the summary must include:
   a. The patient's problem list along with pertinent history, physical, and laboratory information.
   b. Plans: therapy, scheduled consults, medications, other follow-up needs.

4. If the prisoner is to be released from custody, the discharge summary must include all of the information described in Section III.H.3. Additionally, the patient should be given a copy of the discharge summary with copies of all pertinent laboratory and diagnostic tests to give their new providers necessary clinical information.

5. Correctional health care providers should work with government and non-government health care agencies to develop referral criteria and programs to ensure continuity of care for discharged prisoners with significant health care needs including medications and supportive care.

6. Prisoners discharged from custody must be given a supply of essential medications that is sufficient for at least 2 weeks or until they may reasonably be expected to obtain necessary community-based follow-up care. The medications must be packaged in containers labeled according to state pharmaceutical standards.

7. Discharge planning should include assisting eligible prisoners to enroll in insurance programs prior to their release to facilitate their continuity of care. These programs would include: Medicaid, Medicare, special adolescent health insurance programs, or disease specific programs such as the Ryan White program.

Cross Reference

Chronic Care Management, IV

Chapter IV ⸻

Chronic Care Management ⸻

Principle: Jails and prisons must have a system in place to manage patients with chronic medical diseases. While health care staff must work within the security arrangements of the jail or prison, they must also identify any impediments of the security system that make chronic care management difficult or impossible. Incarceration must not compromise appropriate chronic disease management.

Public Health Rationale: To prevent morbidity and mortality of incarcerated persons with chronic disease, jails and prisons must have a system in place to appropriately treat chronic diseases.

Satisfactory Compliance:

The components of a chronic disease management system must include the following:

1. The ability to identify prisoners with chronic disease at intake and to diagnose patients with new-onset disease in the general population. In both jails and prisons, persons with chronic disease must be identified at intake. This requires appropriate intake screening by health care providers who are capable of taking a complete history and in making an initial assessment of the patient. Required medical treatments, including medication, HIV therapy, oncological chemotherapy, and other required treatments, must be promptly re-instituted. Early physician examination and review of the patient is important. For many disease categories, (e.g., diabetes, coronary artery disease, cancer, etc.) a physician should examine the patient as part of the first day intake process. Licensed and trained staff must be available to make periodic health assessments and examinations of persons for episodic care so that new-onset chronic disease can be diagnosed. These periodic health assessments should stress screening for those chronic diseases with high prevalence in the age and sex group of the examined individual.

2. The ability to track prisoners with chronic disease by disease category and by housing location when prisoners are moved or transferred within the correctional system. Prisoners frequently change housing assignments or are

transferred between facilities. Changing prisoner housing assignments within a correctional system, or poor record keeping systems, may result in losing patients to follow up their chronic disease. Therefore, there must be a system in place to identify chronic disease patients if they are transferred within the correctional system. Additionally, problem lists and separate chronic disease lists that identify chronic disease patients by disease category must be available.

3. An appointment scheduling system that ensures regular follow-up of patients with chronic disease at appropriate intervals. There must be a system in place that permits regular medical appointment scheduling for persons with chronic disease. Appointments should be scheduled quarterly or more frequently if clinically required. Appointment scheduling must remain continuous if a prisoner changes housing assignment. Appointment scheduling must also identify the reason for the medical appointment.

4. A medication delivery system that guarantees prisoners will receive chronic disease medication as directed by the prescribing physician or prescribing provider without interruption. Persons with a chronic disease must obtain prescribed medication in a timely and continuous manner. A system for prescription-based medication delivery must also be in place. Such a system should guarantee that medications are delivered on time and in the manner indicated by the prescription. Pill line arrangements must be scheduled in a manner that corresponds with the time intervals recommended for the ingestion of medication. When medications are required to be taken at certain intervals to be effective, and these time intervals do not correspond to scheduled pill calls, then special arrangements must be made to ensure the prisoner takes the medication on time. A system must also be in place to renew medication for patients with chronic disease and to ensure a continuous supply of medication.

5. Application of contemporary standards of care in treatment of patients with chronic disease by practitioners who are qualified by certification or training. Protocols for treatment of chronic diseases in the jails and prisons must be based on contemporary national standards of community care. Adherence to protocols must be monitored for compliance. Treatment of HIV disease should be conducted by physicians with specific expertise in treating this infection.

Examples of contemporary standards of care include:
a. *Standards of Medical Care for Patients with Diabetes Mellitus*, American Diabetic Association.
b. *Expert Panel Report 2: Guidelines for the Diagnosis and Management of Asthma*, National Heart Lung and Blood Institute.
c. *The Sixth Report of the Joint National Committee on Prevention, Detection, Evaluation and Treatment of High Blood Pressure*, National Heart Lung and Blood Institute.
d. *Second Report on Detection, Evaluation and Treatment of High Blood Cholesterol*, National Cholesterol Education Project.
e. *Guidelines for the Use of Antiretroviral Agents in HIV-Infected Adults and Adolescents*, Centers for Disease Control and Prevention (CDC).

6. Monitoring of chronic disease treatment outcomes to achieve continuously improved care. Satisfactory management of patients with chronic diseases is evidenced by measured outcomes. Examples of measurable indicators of onsite outcomes may include:
   a. Average hemoglobin A1c of all patients with diabetes;
   b. Percent of patients with diabetes who have dilated fundoscopy on a yearly basis to diagnose and manage retinopathy;
   c. Percent of patients with diabetes who are tested annually for microalbuminuria;
   d. Percent of patients with HIV infection who are candidates for anti-retroviral therapy who have undetectable viral loads;
   e. Percent of patients with HIV infection and CD4 counts below 200 who are on pneumocystis pneumonia prophylaxis;
   f. Percent of patients with hypertension who are under control (e.g., blood pressure less than 140/90);
   g. Percent of females who have annual cervical cytologies (Pap tests); and
   h. Percent of patients with hyperlipidemia who have LDL cholesterol within the National Cholesterol Education Project's risk stratified goal.

   These examples should change as standards of care change. In addition to outcome measures of onsite care, all emergency room visits, hospitalizations, and deaths should be reviewed as sentinel events. These events should be reviewed to see whether chronic disease management inadequacies contributed to the resultant morbidity or mortality. The team of individuals (e.g., physician, nurse practitioner, or physician assistant, nurse) who care for the patient with chronic disease should analyze outcome data and sentinel events to correct any system problems or individual patient treatment plans that may affect outcome results.

7. Management of patients with chronic illness must include subspecialty referral and diagnostic evaluation as indicated by the condition of the patient. When an illness is not responding to usual management at the jail or prison, consultation with a specialty care practitioner must be provided. Other diagnostic evaluations must be provided as indicated by the condition of the patient. Some patients with chronic disease will need diagnostic studies (e.g., cardiac catheterization or radiologic procedures) that may not be available onsite. These subspecialty consultations or diagnostic studies must be performed in a timely fashion consistent with national contemporary disease management standards in the community. When the jail or prison does not have the ability to provide for appropriate care for a prisoner (e.g., advanced nursing skill needs) the prisoner must be transferred to a medical facility where appropriate care can be provided.

8. Patient education to improve self care skills and compliance with treatment. Peer education is an important part of this. Peer support groups to facilitate understanding and reinforce importance with compliance should be encouraged.

Cross References

Initial Medical Screening and Complete Medical Examination, III.A

Follow-Up, III.C
Periodic Health Assessment, III.G
Wellness Promotion and Health Education, IX

References

Puisis M, Robertson, JM. Chronic disease management. In: *Clinical Practice in Correctional Medicine.* Puisis M, ed. St. Louis, Mo: Mosby Publishers; 1998.

MacFarlane IA. The development of healthcare services for diabetic prisoners. *Postgrad Med J.* 1996;72:214-217.

Legal References

Feliciano v Gonzalez, 13 F Supp 2d 151 (DPR 1998).
Madrid v Gomez, 889 F Supp 1146 (ND Ca 1995).
Kaminsky v Rosenblum, 738 F Supp 1309 (SD NY 1990).
Inmates of Occoquan v Barry, 717 F Supp 854, 867-868 (DDC 1989).
Tillery v Owens, 719 F Supp 1256, 1308-1309 (WD Pa 1989).

Mental Health Services ─────────────────

V.A PROVISION OF CONTINUUM OF CARE

Principle: Mental health services, both diagnostic and therapeutic, must be made available to all incarcerated persons with acute and/or chronic psychiatric disorders including behavioral and emotional conditions, substance use disorders, and developmental disabilities.

Public Health Rationale: Incarcerated populations include a disproportionate number of individuals with a history of mental health problems. For example, jail and prison populations have a high prevalence rate of psychiatric disorders, drug and alcohol abuse, and co-morbid neurological disorders. In addition, incarceration may cause the onset of psychiatric disorders and/or exacerbate current or pre-existing psychiatric disorders. Suicide is a leading cause of death for incarcerated persons, with the highest rate found in jails. Individuals with undiagnosed or untreated psychiatric disorders suffer disproportionately within prisons and jails and are often subject to disciplinary segregation or physical restraint. Furthermore, prisoners with psychiatric disorders are often ostracized and harassed by other prisoners due to psychiatric symptoms or behaviors.

An important component of treatment for people with mental illness is access to mental health programs, medication, and therapy. Supportive housing environments, and not the revolving use of punitive segregation, must allow mentally ill prisoners who are not in need of constant psychiatric observation or treatment to be housed in safe environments where they can participate in day-to-day treatment and supported living programs during incarceration.

Since it is difficult to provide adequate mental health services in jails and prisons, jurisdictions must develop programs for diverting people with mental illnesses from correctional institutions and treat prisoners with mental illness in more appropriate community settings. While diversion programs are critical to the well being of a society, these programs are outside of the scope of these standards for jails and prisons.

Satisfactory Compliance:

1. Every jail and prison must have a plan of care to ensure that the full range of mental health services are available to prisoners who need them to treat current symptoms, prevent further deterioration, and promote good mental health. Provision of mental health services to prisoners must be consistent with national community standards for the delivery of mental health care and with all other sections of these standards.

2. There must be written policies and procedures for mental health services that are available to prisoners. A written description of these services and policies must be given to each prisoner upon admission and must be available in the prisoners' primary languages. If the prisoner is illiterate or unable to read due to a functional impairment, this information should be read and explained to the prisoner. Copies of these written policies and procedures must be posted in public areas and additional copies should be made available to prisoners upon request.

3. Every jail and prison mental health program must have the following components and programs with accompanying written policies and procedures detailing the services provided:

   a. **Means of accessing mental health services**

      (1) *Screening and assessment at intake:* There must be psychiatric screening and assessment for each prisoner admitted to jail or prison by an independent licensed mental health provider or a properly trained independent health care provider to evaluate the prisoner for acute and/or chronic psychiatric disorders and/or the need for immediate psychiatric intervention for individuals with acute and/or severe conditions, such as psychosis, delirium, or suicide risk. This screening must include:

         (*a*) Assessment regarding the need for special housing or services, such as mental observation housing, suicide watch, immediate treatment, or transfer to a psychiatric hospital. The jail or prison must have special housing and services available onsite. In small jails without special housing capability, arrangements must be made with the closest appropriate local psychiatric facility where a prisoner can be immediately transported.

         (*b*) Evaluation for withdrawal and detoxification from alcohol and drugs. Health care staff must also screen for drug and alcohol withdrawal during the initial medical screening;

         (*c*) When intake screening is performed by appropriately trained independent licensed health care providers, prisoners deemed in need of mental health and/or substance abuse treatment services should be referred to mental health staff.

         (*d*) If the facility does not have mental health staff onsite, independent licensed health care providers must be responsible for taking appropriate measures to stabilize the patient until a complete mental health evaluation can be performed. These measures may include referral of the patient to a hospital, or placing the patient in an appropriately designed and admin-istered mental observation area (with or without suicide watch), or in an infirmary or medical holding area with an adequate number of staff, clinical knowledge, and resources.

(e) Prisoners identified as having mental health problems at intake must be referred to and receive follow-up care by the facility mental health service in accordance with these standards.

(2) *Crisis intervention and management:* There must be specific poli-cies and procedures regarding crisis intervention and management of acute psychiatric episodes including, but not limited to, psy-chotic behaviors, suicidal ideation, gestures or attempts, and anxi-ety disorders including panic attacks. Management should include emergency medication protocols appropriate for each disorder, one to one and/or close observation areas with appropriate staffing, and therapy or counseling as appropriate. Where seclusion and/or restraints are necessary for the safety of the prisoner or clinical staff, the formal guidelines outlined in Section VIII must be followed. Policies and procedures must address and include the following:

(a) Crisis intervention services for the management of acute psy-chiatric symptoms must be available to prisoners. In facilities where independent licensed mental health providers are onsite around-the-clock, it is the responsibility of the mental health staff to respond to prisoners in acute emotional or mental dis-tress.

(b) If the facility does not have 24-hour-a-day mental health staffing, formal procedures and protocols must be in place for health care staff to respond to emergencies and to assess the need for further intervention. The jail or prison must have formal arrange-ments with one or more local, offsite psychiatric agencies or licensed professionals to provide mental health crisis inter-vention and management services on an around-the-clock basis. In such cases, an independent licensed mental health provider (ILMHP) must be able to evaluate and treat the prisoner with-in one hour of being contacted, regardless of whether trans-port of the prisoner or the crisis management team is involved. Specific written protocols and agreements must describe the process for obtaining services.

(c) Emergency and urgent psychiatric treatment provided within prisons and jails must be consistent with current recommen-dations for community-based care developed by the American Psychiatric Association, American Psychological Association, the American Association of Emergency Psychiatry, and other national organizations that develop and monitor standards of mental health treatment in community settings.

(d) Involuntary emergency treatment must be in line with state mental health laws regulating emergency psychiatric treatment and these standards.

(3) *Referral or self-referral of prisoner:* Prisoners should be referred to the mental health system by mental health or health care staff on the basis of the intake screening or at any other time when the need for such services are identified, by health care, custodial and other correctional staff, or by prisoners themselves. Prisoners must be seen as soon as possible by an independent licensed mental health care provider (no later than 72 hours after receipt of the referral). Services must include:

   (a) A brief or extended evaluation/assessment must be conducted by an independent licensed mental health provider. The evaluation or assessment need not be performed by a psychiatrist as long as one is available for consultation.

   (b) An individualized treatment plan must be developed to direct and assess the effectiveness of the treatment provided to the prisoner. The scope of the plan will differ with the intensity of the services required, but every prisoner evaluated by mental health providers who is deemed in need of any mental health care or follow-up must have a treatment plan.

b. **Special housing:** In addition to the services provided in the mental health clinic, each correctional facility must be able to provide the following levels of mental health care that involve special housing facilities and staffing either onsite or through an agreement with an outside licensed provider:

   (Note: Some correctional systems may further differentiate the levels of care beyond the two levels described in these standards. This is fine as long as the levels of care are accompanied by appropriate levels and numbers of staff and are consistent with the principles and standards articulated in these standards and national standards of community-based care.)

   (1) *Level I:* Onsite special observation housing unit

      (a) PURPOSE: To provide prisoners diagnosed with psychiatric disorders a protected living unit with daily mental health staff presence and easy access to day-to-day treatment and outpatient-type mental health treatment. This type of intervention helps prevent further mental health deterioration, victimization, and punitive intervention. This unit should be used if there is a clinically determined need for mental health observation to clarify diagnostic or behavioral risk issues. This level of service is not appropriate for prisoners who are in crisis or need 24-hour-a-day observation or oversight by mental health staff; are imminently suicidal; or in need of seclusion, forced medication, or restraint. This unit is not for persons who require aggressive stabilization on neuroleptics or for anyone with acute medical needs.

      The special observation housing unit can serve as a transitional unit for prisoners who have spent time in an inpatient psychiatric unit or a Level II unit (as described below), but are not yet ready for general population housing within the jail or prison. These units are places within the jail or prison where prisoners with serious mental illness or developmental disabilities can be housed safely (safe from victimization as well as safe from the likelihood of getting into disciplinary difficulty and being sent to punitive segregation) for transitional periods or for the duration of their incarceration.

(b) ADMISSION AND DISCHARGE

    (i)   Prisoners should be admitted to the special observation housing unit for protection, observation, stabilization, psychiatric evaluation, and short-term treatment of psychiatric and substance abuse disorders where the prisoner requires a supportive environment, but does not need intensive psychiatric services.

    (ii) Prisoners should only be admitted following initial assessment by mental health staff or an independent licensed health care provider (in the absence of mental health staff onsite at the time of the admission).

    (iii) Prisoners housed in the observation unit must be evaluated by an independent licensed mental health provider within 48 hours of admission to the unit (or sooner as the condition demands). This provider, in conjunction with the treatment team, should be responsible for determining the prisoner's further treatment needs and aftercare placement and should develop an initial treatment plan. Such determination may involve continued observation onsite in an observation unit or a unit with more extensive mental health staffing, transfer to a licensed psychiatric facility, or discharge to general population housing.

    (iv) No prisoner should be discharged from the special observation unit without an evaluation by an independent licensed mental health provider. However, prisoners on this unit may be transferred to a higher level of care by other mental health or health care staff in consultation with a psychiatrist in emergency situations. Decisions to admit or discharge prisoners from this or any other health care or mental health care unit must never be made by non-clinical staff or correctional staff.

(c) STAFFING

    (i)   Staffing in observation units must be sufficient to allow for observation of all patients by correctional staff who have been specially trained to work on these units. In addition, there must be sufficient mental health staff to allow for daily meetings with unit residents and sufficient number of staff to provide other therapeutic time as required by the individual treatment plans.

(ii)   Unit mental health staff should make daily rounds with an independent licensed mental health provider to assess mental status, appropriateness of the housing placement, treatment response, and need for continued observation for unit patients. Rounds must be made with a psychiatrist at least once each week.

(iii)   Prisoners housed in the observation unit will be re-evaluated on a weekly basis by a member of the mental health staff and bi-weekly by a psychiatrist.

(iv)   Custody staff working in the special observation unit must complete specialized training and demonstrate competency in the appropriate monitoring and management of patients with cognitive, behavioral, and developmental disorders.

(v)   Unit clinical staff are responsible for the maintenance of the therapeutic environment, including training of unit clinical and custody staff as needed.

(*d*) PROGRAM

(i)   Therapeutic interventions used in the observation units should include, but not be limited to, individual and group therapy, crisis counseling, and administration of psychotropic medications per guidelines described in these standards and consistent with national standards for community care in outpatient settings.

(ii)   Physical and chemical restraints should not be used in this setting. However, structured mental health observation should be used. Any prisoner believed to be in need of physical restraint or forced medication must be evaluated by a psychiatrist in accordance with these standards and be moved safely to a Level II facility (if one exists in the jail or prison), with the limitations listed in the following section on Level II units, or to an offsite licensed psychiatric facility.

(iii)   Prisoners admitted to the observation unit will have full access to programming within the institution.

(2) *Level II:* Onsite psychiatric treatment unit

(*a*) PURPOSE: The psychiatric treatment unit has the capacity to function as an acute diversion unit, a psychiatric emergency service, and a unit for prisoners in need of intensive psychiatric services who do not requite acute psychiatric hospitalization. This level of care is appropriate for prisoners who need intensive psychiatric treatment, frequent doses of psychiatric medication, and frequent observation by mental health and nursing staff. This level of care is not a hospital setting and cannot offer seclusion, restraints beyond 8 hours, or forced medication (except on an emergency basis, and only then in accordance with state and local laws and these standards).

(*b*) ADMISSION AND DISCHARGE

    (i)   Prisoners thought to be in need of intensive mental health services must be evaluated by an independent licensed mental health provider (e.g., psychiatrist, psychologist, psychiatric nurse, or psychiatric social worker) within 2 hours of referral to the unit and, if deemed in need of intensive mental health services, must be admitted to a psychiatric treatment unit. If one is not available within the institution, the prisoner must be transferred to a licensed offsite psychiatric unit or hospital. Only independent licensed mental health providers may admit people to a psychiatric treatment unit.

    (ii)   Such consultation must include an in-person mental health evaluation provided onsite. There must be no exception for weekends and holidays.

    (iii)   An onsite psychiatric treatment unit must offer intensive psychiatric treatment for severe psychiatric symptomatology, behavioral disorders, and behavior or ideation that indicates a potential for danger to self or others.

    (iv)   Only a psychiatrist may discharge a patient from this unit and only to a suitable unit or facility.

(*c*) STAFFING

    (i)   There must be 24-hour psychiatric staff coverage by nurses and other health professionals trained in therapeutic approaches and interventions with individuals with psychiatric, behavioral, and developmental disorders. There must be psychiatrists on call around-the-clock who can respond to any emergencies that arise onsite. There must be sufficient onsite psychiatric coverage each day to ensure adequate time for consultation with patients and supervision. Staff must have training and experience equivalent to mental health professionals providing this type of psychiatric care within comparable psychiatric settings in the community and constant, including arms-length observation of patients who are suicidal or present a danger to self or others. Units will follow standards for training, staffing and protocols required by JCAHO and/or the state mental health authority for comparable levels of care for such sites in the community.

    (ii)   Independent licensed mental health providers must make daily rounds to assess mental status, appropriateness of the housing, treatment response, and need for continued observation.

    (iii)   Independent licensed mental health providers must be responsible for the development and maintenance of the therapeutic environment as well as the training of the custody staff.

       (iv) For each prisoner, a weekly clinical treatment case review must occur with a unit treatment team that includes the psychiatrist, other mental health providers, and nursing staff. As appropriate, the meeting should include custody staff, social service providers, and the patient. If non-clinical staff are present, the prisoner's confidentiality rights must be protected.

  (d) PROGRAM

       (i)   Prisoners admitted to the unit should be provided with a full psychiatric evaluation to determine the most appropriate interventions to alleviate symptoms, prevent further deterioration, and optimize mental health.

       (ii)   Additional evaluation and intervention will be made available and include psychological testing and behavioral developmental assessment.

       (iii) Interventions that are used in this setting include group and individual psychotherapy, crisis counseling, and appropriate therapeutic use of psychotropic medications. These interventions and the guidelines, standards, and protocols must be consistent with national community standards of care as described in Section V.C and elsewhere in these standards.

       (iv) Physical and involuntary chemical restraints should not be routinely used in onsite psychiatric treatment units. Rather, structured mental health observation should be used. Prisoners in need of physical restraint beyond 8 hours or forced medications beyond an initial dose must be transferred to a licensed psychiatric facility or a psychiatric unit at a licensed and JCAHO accredited hospital.

       (v)   Prisoners admitted to the psychiatric unit will have access to internal programming (e.g., occupational therapy, educational programming, and art therapy) that complements treatment.

       (vi) Based upon the clinical assessment and the treatment plan, prisoners may have access to some or all institutional programs as determined by the treatment team, such as school or vocational programs.

(3) *Level III:* Acute psychiatric hospitalization:

In the event that a psychiatric unit (Level II and above) is not available within the jail or prison and the prisoner requires Level III psychiatric care, transfer to a facility outside of the institution must take place. In addition, all prisoners who require involuntary administration of psychotropic medication beyond an initial dose and/or who require seclusion, and/or restraints for psychiatric purposes for more than 8 hours must be transferred to an offsite hospital for psychiatric care. Formal written agreements must be established with a hospital or psychiatric facility that is licensed and JCAHO accredited.

(a) ADMISSION AND DISCHARGE

    (i)   The decision to transfer a prisoner to a psychiatric facility outside of the institution must be made by a psychiatrist who has examined the prisoner and has determined the need for inpatient psychiatric treatment.

    (ii)   In facilities where a psychiatrist is not onsite or available on an emergency basis, an ILMHP may authorize such a transfer. Where no ILMHP is onsite or available, the facility must have written agreements with a licensed mental health facility that can receive psychiatric emergencies within an hour's notice for appropriate assessment and admission.

    (iii)   If transfer is not immediately practical, the prisoner may receive emergency psychotropic medication according to procedures consistent with these standards and state law when the patient is transferred to an offsite psychiatric facility.

    (iv)   Involuntary administration of psychotropic medications should be administered only in psychiatric settings where experienced mental health clinicians are available for observation and intervention.

(b) THERAPEUTIC MODALITIES AND PROGRAM: A therapeutic program should be available based on the individual needs of the prisoner-patient consistent with national community standards of mental health care and those required by the accrediting and licensing body and are beyond the scope of these standards regarding jail and prison-based care.

c. **Psychiatric screening prior to and during placement in punitive segregation**

    (1) Psychiatric screening and assessment of prisoners prior to placement in punitive segregation must be performed to ensure that those with serious psychiatric disorders are not placed in punitive segregation or are appropriately treated.

    (2) Any prisoner who has a history of significant mental illness, or is at risk of committing suicide, or displays any signs of significant mental illness, must not be placed in punitive segregation.

    (3) Prisoners who are in punitive segregation must be assessed a minimum of one month after confinement and then at least every 3 months thereafter (more frequently if indicated by prisoner request, custodial identification, health care/mental health provider request, or if psychiatric signs are apparent) for the development of psychiatric disorders.

    (4) Segregated prisoners must be removed from the punitive segregation cell to a private office where confidentiality is protected to be

            assessed by a psychiatrist or other independent licensed mental health professional.

     (5) If a prisoner requires assessment due to onset of psychiatric symptoms, an emergency referral must be made and the prisoner must be seen promptly.

   d. **Suicide prevention program** (See Section V.B.E)

   e. **Discharge planning** (See Section III.H, Transfer and Discharge)

Legal References

Doty v County of Lassen, 37 F3d 540, 546 (9th Cir 1994).

Greason v Kemp, 891 F2d 829, 834 (11th Cir 1990).

Smith v Jenkins, 919 F2d 90, 92-93 (8th Cir 1990).

Langley v Coughlin, 888 F2d 252, 254 (2nd Cir 1989).

Waldrop v Evans, 871 F2d 1030, 1033 (11th Cir), *rehearing denied*, 880 F2d 421 (11th Cir 1989).

Eng v Smith, 849 F2d 80, 82 (2nd Cir 1988).

Cortes-Quinones v Jiminez-Nettleship, 842 F2d 556 (1st Cir 1988).

Rogers v Evans, 792 F2d 1953, 1058 (11th Cir 1986).

Wellman v Faulkner, 715 F2d 269, 272 (7th Cir 1983), *cert. denied*, 468 US 1217, 104 S Ct 3587, 82 L Ed 2d 885 (1984).

Hoptowit v Ray, 682 F2d 1237, 1253 (9th Cir 1982).

Ramos v Lamm, 639 F2d 559, 574 (10th Cir 1980), *cert. denied*, 450 US1041, 101 S Ct 1759, 68 L Ed. 2d 239 (1981).

Inmates of Allegheny County Jail v Pierce, 612 F2d 754, 763 (3rd Cir 1979).

Bowring v Godwin, 551 F2d 44, 47-48 (4th Cir 1977).

Perri v Coughlin, No 90-CV-1160 (ND NY 1999).

Feliciano v Gonzalez, 13 F Supp 2d 151 (DPR 1998).

Hartman ex. rel. Esate of Douglas v Correctional Medical Services, 960 F Supp 1577 (MD Fla 1996).

Viero v Bufano, 925 F Supp 1374 (ND Ill 1996).

Coleman v Wilson, 912 F Supp 1282 (ED Ca 1995).

Arnold on behalf of HB v Lewis, 803 F Supp 246, 257 (D Ariz 1992).

Tillery v Owens, 719 F Supp 1256, 1303-1304 (WD Pa 1989), *aff'd* 907 F2d 418 (3rd Cir 1990).

Inmates of Occoquan v Barry, 717 F Supp 854, 868 (DDC 1989).

Balla v Idaho State Bd. of Correction, 595 F Supp 1558, 1579 (D Idaho 1984), *modified on other grounds* 869 F2d 461(9th Cir 1988).

Ruiz v Estelle, 503 F Supp 1265, 1339 (SD Tex 1980), *aff'd in part and rev'd in part*, 679F2d 1115 (5th Cir 1982).

V.B   PRINCIPLES OF CARE

A.   Services Must Not Be Imposed

    Principle: The state should not mandate treatment for any prisoner unless it has been determined by an independent licensed mental health provider that a prisoner, by reason of mental disability, poses a clear and present danger of grave injury to himself (including exacerbation of symptoms by pathologically-based refusal of treatment) or to others. The precise language should be determined by each state's standard for civil commitment. Only then should intervention be mandated and then with the least restrictive measures: (a) in response to an emergency; or (b) on a continuing basis, only after civil judicial direction by the appropriate court after the prisoner has been afforded an independent psychiatric evaluation; and (c) such continuing mandated treatment should be provided only in a licensed acute psychiatric facility or a psychiatric unit of a hospital in the community where the protections of due process safeguards available as required by the jurisdiction.

Public Health Rationale: Health professionals do not have the legal or ethical right to impose treatment on an individual unless there is a clear and present threat to the public or to the individual. If, by virtue of mental disorder, the well-being of the public is threatened, the public, including the individual who is mentally disordered, must be protected. At the same time, the mentally ill have the right to appropriate treatment or, under certain circumstances, to refuse treatment as long as their civil rights and their right to due process is protected.

Satisfactory Compliance:

1. Each jail and prison must provide onsite ambulatory and inpatient psychiatric and substance abuse treatment or they must provide prisoners, through formal subcontracts, with such services at one or more licensed mental health facilities.

2. Involuntary treatment, hospitalization, or medication of a prisoner who is posing a clear present threat to self or others may take place only in accordance with state law and with written procedures and under the following conditions:

   a. Only the least restrictive measures necessary to respond to an emergency should be used. The specific reasons for the intervention chosen should be documented in the patient's record and should be reviewed as part of supervision and quality improvement;

   b. These measures must be used only with a written order from a psychiatrist who has evaluated the patient. If a psychiatrist is not onsite (and the patient cannot be safely transported to an offsite hospital), an independent licensed mental health or trained health care provider may administer the emergency medications or treatment. The patient must then be seen by a psychiatrist within 1 hour or transferred to a hospital;

   c. The responsible physician must document in the patient's chart the patient's condition, the threat posed, the reason for the proposed intervention, and the length of the period of the proposed intervention;

   d. An order to treat against a prisoner's will should be valid for no longer than 24 hours or for a period permitted by state law, whichever is shorter;

   e. No prisoner should receive involuntary psychiatric treatment without a prior evaluation and a written order by a psychiatrist. Prisoners' right to due process must be observed;

   f. If involuntary treatment is indicated beyond the first 24 hours, further treatment should take place only in a licensed offsite psychiatric or fully accredited inpatient setting. Under no circumstances should a prisoner treated against his will remain in a jail or prison that does not have 24-hour staffing by independent licensed mental health providers.

3. Mental health treatment should not be used as a reward, privilege, or punishment.

4. Psychiatric and mental health services should be provided on a voluntary basis for psychiatric disorders as diagnosed by an independent licensed mental health provider.

5. Psychotropic medication should only be prescribed with the informed consent of the prisoner, except in emergency situations.

B.   Professional Independence: Separation of Functions

Principle: Mental health professionals must separate functions to maintain professional independence and protect the therapeutic relationship. For example, mental health professionals who participate in administrative decision-making processes, such as parole and furlough must not provide direct therapeutic services for those prisoners. Treating professionals must not compromise the therapeutic relationship by assuming a role in the decision-making process regarding release. However, mental health providers must assert their protective function with regard to housing and security of prisoners, such as keeping them out of housing situations that would cause deterioration.

Public Health Rationale: The intent of this principle is to protect the therapeutic relationship. The therapeutic relationship is inevitably affected by the patient's knowledge of the therapist's potential role in rewarding or sanctioning the prisoner.

Satisfactory Compliance:

1. Mental health providers must explain to the prisoner at the outset of therapy that they will not contribute to the decision-making process of any administrative board (e.g., parole, work release, or furlough) or allow themselves to be obligated by correctional administration to do so. In specific instances, the therapist, with the consent of the prisoner, may make available relevant opinion or data for the decision-making process or act as the prisoner's advocate.

2. Mental health providers who treat prisoners must not sit on parole boards. Whenever a parole board determines that input is needed regarding the mental health of a prisoner, that information must be provided by a mental health provider who is not treating the prisoner. Only with permission from the patient may the non-treating mental health provider consult the medical record or interview the patient.

3. There must be clear and formal procedures in the jail or prison for resolving disputes between custody and mental health staff regarding custody issues, appropriateness of housing, and discipline when there are significant mental health consequences of such decisions (e.g., determinations that a person cannot be housed in punitive segregation).

4. Prisoners' need for mental health treatment must take precedence over custody and control procedures if such custody or control procedures would increase the likelihood of suicide or psychiatric deterioration of the prisoner. There must be specific written protocols describing the procedure for making these decisions.

5. Determination of competency and criminal responsibility must be addressed by court-appointed mental health professionals who are not working for the jail- or prison-based mental health program. Although mental health providers

in the jail or prison are normally not involved in forensic decisions, exceptions may exist when the treating professional believes that the issue of a
detainee's incompetence to stand trial is not being addressed.

C. Confidentiality

Principle: Full confidentiality of all information obtained in the course of psychiatric treatment should be maintained at all times except when legal and professional obligations require mental health professionals to respond to a clear and
present danger of grave injury to the prisoner or others or if the prisoner intends to
escape.

Public Health Rationale: Mental health providers who treat prisoners have an
ethical and professional responsibility to protect prisoner confidentiality.
Confidentiality is an essential component of the therapeutic relationship. Moreover,
effective mental health treatment cannot be conducted unless patients have confi-
dence in the protection of the information they reveal.

Satisfactory Compliance:

1. In all therapeutic relationships, the mental health provider must explain the
   parameters of confidentiality, including the degree to which this guarantee
   extends and a precise delineation of its limits prior to beginning treatment.
   Exceptions include, but may not be limited to, those noted above (e.g., the
   mental health provider must abide by mandatory state child abuse reporting requirements or the duty to warn and/or protect an individual threatened by a patient). These parameters should be periodically reviewed with
   the prisoner.

2. Prisoners who reveal information to a mental health provider that falls outside the limits of confidentiality must be told, prior to disclosure by the
   provider, that such information will be disclosed. If the mental health provider
   believes that informing the prisoner of intent to disclose information will
   increase the likelihood of grave injury to the prisoner or others, the provider
   may delay informing the prisoner of that disclosure.

3. The limits or boundaries of confidentiality must be consistent with applicable state laws for the non-incarcerated population. Mental health data
   must be entered into the health care records and be handled in accordance
   with the provisions of the Health Care Records section of these standards.
   The mental health data must be restricted to the facts of treatment, diagnosis, prognosis, treatment plan, and medication. Sensitive or highly personal data must not be included in the health care record, but may be kept in
   separate notes maintained by the provider. (Note: Such notes, typically called
   process notes, can be subpoenaed by the court as part of the medical record
   and are not necessarily protected under doctor/patient confidentiality).

4. While ensuring the safety of mental health treatment staff (e.g., through visual observation by custody staff), all interviews and treatment sessions will
   be conducted in a confidential setting with auditory privacy.

Legal References

Vitek v Jones, 445 US 480, 494-496, 100 S Ct 1254 (1980).

Buckley v Rogerson, 133 F3d 1125 (8th Cir 1998).
Coleman v Wilson, 912 F Supp 1282 (ED Ca1995).
Burks v Teasdale, 492 F Supp 650, 679 (WD Mo 1980).
Eckerhart v Hensley, 475 F Supp 908 (WD Mo 1979).
Negron v Preiser, 382 F Supp 535, 543 (SD NY 1974).

D. Therapeutic Services

Principle: A comprehensive range of psychiatric services must be provided to prisoners and should include treatment modalities and services commonly used within mental health treatment settings in the community. Because of the significant variability in mental health system capacity within and across states, such treatments and services must include those that have demonstrated effectiveness (i.e., evidence-based) such as those outlined in the Surgeon General's Report on Mental Illness, the Surgeon General's Report on Suicide Prevention, and the Schizophrenia PORT study as well as those promoted by national professional organizations (e.g., American Psychiatric Association, American Psychological Association, American Association of Child and Adolescent Psychiatrists, American Association of Community Psychiatrists). Such practice guidelines, treatment protocols, and standards should be adopted and adapted as needed in order to ensure the provision of adequate, appropriate, and comprehensive psychiatric and mental health care for jail and prison populations.

Public Health Rationale: All prisoners have the right to comprehensive psychiatric and mental health services with the goal of alleviating and minimizing the development of emotional and mental suffering and impairment. Voluntary therapy, treatments, and services that prevent decompensation, exacerbation, and /or recurrence of symptoms, and promote and sustain prisoner recovery at all levels of care should be provided. Such interventions may also assist prisoners in preparing to cope more effectively with the stress of incarceration and with the re-adjustment to community life post-release.

Satisfactory Compliance:

1. Jails and prisons must have the capability (i.e., staff, space, and resources) to provide the mental health program services described in section V of these standards. Such services should include, but not be limited to: psychodynamic, behavioral, cognitive, and/or other appropriate individual or group therapy modalities; psychosocial and vocational rehabilitation services; and medication management (outlined below). Jails and prisons must have detailed written policies and protocols that describe the elements of the mental health service and that are consistent with national standards for mental health care in the community. In particular, the following must be provided:

   a. **Psychotherapy and counseling**
      (1) Prisoners with psychiatric diagnoses should be assessed to determine the most appropriate therapeutic intervention, including group or family therapy;
      (2) Individual and group psychotherapy should be provided by independent licensed mental health providers who have demonstrated competency and appropriate credentials. Therapy and coun-

seling services may also be provided by other properly trained and credentialed mental health professionals. Individual and group therapy services should be supervised by a psychiatrist or a clinical psychologist with demonstrated experience and expertise in individual and group psychotherapy, except in cases where another mental health provider has appropriate specialty training, credentials, and experience regarding a particular modality.

b. **Psychotropic medication.** Policies regarding the use of psychotropic medication must address the following:

(1) Psychotropic medication may be prescribed only by a physician or an ILMHP (as permitted by state law). Psychotropic medication must be prescribed in accordance with generally accepted pharmacological principles and contemporary national standards in the community. In most cases, a psychiatrist prescribes these medications; however, when a non-psychiatrist prescribes a psychotropic medication, the order must be reviewed by a psychiatrist within 72 hours.

(2) There must be laboratory monitoring of any patient placed on psychotropic medication consistent with national community standards of care. Ongoing periodic evaluation of medication effectiveness and presence of side effects must be performed in all cases and be consistent with national community standards of care.

(3) Psychotropic medication may be prescribed only if clinically indicated and only as one element of a treatment plan. It can not take the place of appropriate counseling and/or therapy.

(4) Every prisoner receiving psychotropic medication must be seen and evaluated by a psychiatrist at least once a week until stabilized and at least every 4 weeks thereafter.

(5) Female prisoners must be informed of the potential risks of taking psychotropic medication while pregnant.

(6) Medications may be prescribed only with the patient's informed consent.

Legal References

Smith v Jenkins, 919 F2d 90, 92-93 (8th Cir 1990).

Greason v Kemp, 891 F2d 829, 834 (11th Cir 1990).

Waldrop v Evans, 871 F2d 1030, 1033 (11th Cir), *rehearing denied*, 880 F2d 421 (11th Cir 1989).

Langley v Coughlin, 888 F2d 252, 254 (2nd Cir 1989).

Cortes-Quinones v Jiminez-Nettleship, 842 F2d 556 (1st Cir 1988).

Wellman v Faulkner, 715 F2d 269, 272 (7th Cir 1983), *cert. denied*, 468 US 1217 (1984).

Ramos v Lamm, 639 F2d 559, 574 (10th Cir 1980), *cert. denied*, 450 US 1041 (1981).

Feliciano v Gonzalez, 13 F Supp 2d 151 (DPR 1998).

Casey v Lewis, 834 F Supp 1477 (D Ariz 1993).

Arnold on behalf of HB v Lewis, 803 F Supp 246, 257 (D Ariz 1992).

Balla v Idaho State Bd. of Correction, 595 F Supp 1558, 1579 (D Idaho 1984), *modified on other grounds* 869 F2d 461 (9th Cir 1988).

E.　Suicide Prevention

Principal: Jails and prisons must have a suicide prevention program that has written protocols and procedures and includes a staff training component. Jail programs must have specific procedures for early assessments.

Public Health Rationale: Suicide is a leading cause of death among persons confined to correctional facilities even though it is largely preventable through a well-functioning mental health program. Prisoners are especially at risk for suicide when first admitted to a jail. For example, 50% of jail suicides occur in the first 24 hours and 27% occur during the first 3 hours after admission. Health and custody staff must be trained to recognize warning signs of suicidal intent and devise appropriate plans to safeguard life. Whereas correctional authorities have responsibility for safe custody, health staff possess the training and expertise to recognize signs of depression and aberrant behavior such as suicidal intent.

Satisfactory compliance: Elements of an effective suicide prevention program must include the following:

1. Jail and prison health staff with appropriate training must screen prisoners for suicidal intent or ideation as part of the admission medical evaluation;
2. Jail and prison health staff must also screen prisoners for suicidal intent upon transfer to another facility;
3. When an at-risk prisoner is identified by medical staff, the prisoner must be referred to onsite mental health staff (or offsite staff, if mental health staff is not available within the institution) for immediate psychiatric evaluation. Upon mental health evaluation, any prisoner considered to be an imminent suicide risk must be hospitalized on an emergency basis. All other at-risk prisoners must be placed in a mental observation area or treatment unit with a suicide watch (the details of which are dictated by the mental health provider) pending further evaluation by a psychiatrist (within 24 hours);
4. Isolation may increase the chance that a prisoner will commit suicide and must not be used as a substitute for continuity of contact with staff and appropriate supervision. (The practice of placing suicidal prisoners in "safety cells" instead on talking to them and maintaining continuing observation is inappropriate.); and
5. Custody staff must be trained to recognize signs and symptoms of suicidality and there must be written protocols requiring that prisoners be taken immediately to mental health or health care staff (when there is no mental health staff in the facility) whenever (at time of admission or during the course of incarceration) such behavior is observed.

Legal References

Freedman v City of Allentown, 853 F2d 1111, 1115 (3rd Cir 1988).
Estate of Cills v Kaftan, 105 F Supp 2d 391 (D NJ 2000).
Feliciano v Gonzalez, 13 F Supp 2d 151 (DPR 1998).
Viero v Bufano, 925 F Supp 1374 (ND Ill 1996).
Coleman v Wilson, 912 F Supp 1282 (ED Ca 1995).

F.   Specialized Training for Medical and Correctional Personnel

Principle: Medical and correctional personnel must be trained to recognize the signs and symptoms of mental illness. Training must be performed by mental health professionals and be appropriate to the scope of duties of the various staff members.

Public Health Rationale: Prisoners have a high rate of mental and psychiatric illness and are at risk of deterioration or onset of new illness while incarcerated. Properly trained correctional staff can help identify prisoners in need of mental health services and help get prisoners in need of such services to mental health providers within the institution. Medical staff needs special training to identify prisoners in need of mental health services. Prisoners with mental health needs will benefit from having staff specially trained to identify and attend to their needs.

Satisfactory Compliance: Medical and custodial staff must receive training from appropriately trained health and mental health professionals to identify individuals with possible emotional and mental disorders. This training must be part of each employee's orientation and ongoing education must be performed to assure current knowledge of mental health policies and procedures and must include training to recognize (and for medical staff, treatment approaches):

1. Signs and symptoms of mental and emotional disorders prevalent in the prisoner population;
2. Signs of chemical dependence and the symptoms of drug and alcohol intoxication and withdrawal;
3. Adverse reactions to psychotropic medication;
4. Behavioral and cognitive symptoms of developmental disability, especially mental retardation;
5. Potential mental health emergencies and instruction in appropriate intervention in crisis situations;
6. Identification of acute or chronic medical problems of prisoners housed in mental health units;
7. Suicide risk assessment and prevention strategies including procedures for special observation;
8. Instruction in the procedures for referral of prisoners to mental health services for immediate evaluation;
9. Appropriate therapeutic approaches to prevent potentially violent behavior caused by psychiatric disorders, to promote a safe environment, and to integrate specific approaches into the treatment plan; and
10. Training in first aid and CPR by a certified instructor.

G.   Mental Health of Institution

Principle: Mental health professionals should work to enhance the mental health of the institution.

Public Health Rationale: Mental health professionals' training, experience, and expertise can promote healthy mental health functioning for the institutional community.

Satisfactory Compliance: Mental health professionals must:

1. Promote and protect mental health values by consulting regularly with correctional administrators who determine and maintain general policies and procedures;
2. Promote and protect mental health values and offer mental health expertise by using communication skills, group interaction dynamics, or crisis intervention skills. All mental health providers involved in an institutional crisis should be available to:
   a. Act as advisors to prisoner and staff organizations;
   b. Work with correctional personnel in training groups and crisis situations;
   c. Participate in institutional administrative staff meetings;
   d. Consult with any other treatment or service components of the institution, including full participation in quality improvement and utilization review programs; and
   e. Ensure that all institutional staff members are aware of mental health services available and of procedures to refer prisoners seeking or in need of treatment.
3. Monitor the conditions within the correctional setting and intervene proactively (i.e., report and attempt to alleviate) where such conditions jeopardize the mental health of the general population and/or exacerbate the condition of prisoners already suffering from mental illness. Examples of conditions that jeopardize prisoners' mental health include: crowding, excessive heat or cold, cruel or unprofessional behavior by staff, and severe deprivation in solitary confinement settings.

Cross References

Ethical and Legal Issues, I.C
Information Systems, II.A
Staffing and Organization of Health Services, II.C
Initial Medical Screening and Complete Medical Examination, III.A
Transfer and Discharge, III.H
Pharmacy Services, VI.G
Health Services for Women, VII.A
Children and Adolescents, VII.B
Segregation, VII.D
Restraints Administered by Health Care Providers, VIII

References

American Public Health Association. Policy Statement 9929, Diversion from jail for non-violent arrestees with serious mental illness. 1999.

American Public Health Association. Policy Statement 200029, The need for mental health and substance abuse services for the incarcerated mentally ill. 2000.

Cohen F. *The Mentally Disordered Inmate and the Law.* Kingston, NJ: Civic Research Institute; 1998.

Elliott RL. Evaluating the quality of correctional mental health services: an approach to surveying a correctional mental health system. *Behav Sci Law.* 1997;15:427-438.

Felthous AR. Mental health issues in correctional settings. *Behav Sci Law.* 1997;15:379-81.

Fogel CI. Hard time: the stressful nature of incarceration for women. *Issues in Mental Health Nursing.* 1993;14:367-377.

Harmon RB. Mental health and corrections: towards a working partnership. *J Forensic Sci.* 1987;32: 233-241.

Jordan BK, Schlenger WE, Fairbank JA, Caddell JM. Prevalence of psychiatric disorders among incarcerated women: convicted felons entering prison. *Arch Gen Psychiatry.* 1996;53:513-519.

Kaufman E. The violation of psychiatric standards of care in prisons. *Am J Psychiatry.* 1980;137: 566-570.

Metzner JL. An introduction to correctional psychiatry: Part I. *J Am Acad Psychiatry Law.* 1997;25:375-381.

Metzner JL. An introduction to correctional psychiatry: Part II. *J Am Acad Psychiatry Law.* 1997;25:571-579.

Metzner JL. An introduction to correctional psychiatry: Part III. *J Am Acad Psychiatry Law.* 1998;26:107-115.

Metzner JL, Miller RD, Kleinsasser D. Mental health screening and evaluation within prisons. *Bull Am Acad Psychiatry Law.* 1994; 22: 451-457

Metzner JL, Dubovsky SL. The role of the psychiatrist in evaluating a prison mental health system in litigation. *Bull Am Acad Psychiatry Law.* 1986;14:89-95.

Miller RD, Metzner JL. Psychiatric stigma in correctional facilities. *Bull Am Acad Psychiatry Law.* 1994;22:621-628.

Morrison EF. Victimization in prison: implications for the mentally ill inmate and for health professionals. *Arch Psychiatr Nurs.* 1991;5:17-24.

Olivero JM, Roberts JB. Jail suicide and legal redress. *Suicide Life Threat Behav.* 1990;20:138-147.

Pomeroy EC, Kiam R, Abel E. Meeting the mental health needs of incarcerated women. *Health Soc Work.* 1998;23:71-75.

Roskes E, Feldman R. A collaborative community-based treatment program for offenders with mental illness. *Psychiatr Serv.* December 1999; 50:1614-1619.

Teplin LA, Abram KM, McClelland GM. Prevalence of psychiatric disorders among incarcerated women: pretrial jail detainees. *Arch Gen Psychiatry.* 1996;53:505-512.

Legal References

Greason v Kemp, 891 F2d 829, 834 (11th Cir 1990).

Waldrop v Evans, 871 F2d 1030, 1033 (11th Cir), *rehearing denied*, 880 F2d 421 (11th Cir 1989).

Langley v Coughlin, 888 F2d 252, 254 (2nd Cir 1989).

Coleman v Wilson, 912 F Supp 1282 (ED Ca 1995).

Casey v Lewis, 834 F Supp 1477 (D Ariz 1993).

Tillery v Owens, 719 F Supp 1256, 1303-1304 (WD Pa 1989), *aff'd* 907 F2d 418 (3rd Cir 1990).

Feliciano v Gonzalez, 13 F Supp 2d 151 (DPR 1998).

Inmates of Occoquan v Barry, 717 F Supp 854, 868 (DDC 1989).

Burks v Teasdale, 492 F Supp 650, 679 (WD Mo 1980).

Ruiz v Estelle, 503 F Supp 1265, 1339 (SD Tex 1980), *aff'd in part and rev'd in part*, 679 F2d 1115 (5th Cir 1982).

Specific Clinical Issues and Services _____

VI.A COMMUNICABLE DISEASES

Principle: Each prison or jail must have an infection control program that effectively monitors the incidence of infectious and communicable diseases among prisoners and staff, prevents or minimizes the occurrence and transmission of these diseases, and provides individuals with prompt access to prophylactic or therapeutic interventions.

Public Health Rationale: An infection control program ensures the maintenance of a clean and safe healthy environment and decreases the incidence of communicable disease by delineating policies and defining procedures for screening and surveillance systems for early identification of persons with communicable diseases or who are at risk to contract a communicable disease. These programs provide written policies and procedures that assure timely and appropriate intervention for treating the ill and minimizing disease transmission. The CDC is responsible for developing national guidelines for the control of infectious diseases, and their updated recommendations should be the basis of all jail and prison communicable disease policies.

A. Communicable Disease Control

Satisfactory Compliance: Each institution must have written policies and procedures that:

1. Designate a person responsible for the infection control program (position title: Infection Control Coordinator);
2. Create and operate a multi-disciplinary infection control committee that is chaired by the infection control coordinator and that meets regularly to evaluate the policies and procedures of the infection control program, make recommendations for improvement, and address outbreaks or other urgent infectious disease control situations. This committee must:
   a. Include representatives from the administration, medical staff, nursing staff, and other personnel involved in sanitation and the control

of infection (e.g., dietary supervisor, laundry supervisor, environmental health director, and safety officer);

b. Organize and oversee the infection control program and be responsible for infection control policies, procedures, surveillance, and cleaning and disinfectant techniques;

c. Hold meetings on a regular basis and maintain a written record of activities, actions, and recommendations;

d. Develop and update a bloodborne pathogen exposure plan for the prisoners and staff;

e. Develop a protocol for the surveillance and monitoring of communicable diseases within the institution based upon guidelines established by national organizations such as the CDC; and

f. Establish and monitor environmental cleanup procedures and the disposal of infectious materials based upon guidelines established by national organizations such as OSHA and CDC.

3. Oversee the screening, surveillance, and control of infectious and communicable diseases including preventive and control measures specific to the disease and appropriate treatment of identified cases;

4. Maintain the environmental control policies and procedures for the maintenance of a clean, safe, and healthy environment that is in compliance with state and local regulations regarding medical and non-medical waste disposal, water supply, sewage, ventilation, pest control, food handling and preparation, and laundry and housekeeping practices as well as the appropriate education for staff and prisoners to help maintain the institutional environment;

5. Establish policies and procedures for the proper decontamination of medical equipment and the proper disposal of sharps and biohazardous waste;

6. Assure strict adherence to universal precautions by health care workers and others handling blood and body fluids;

7. Maintain communicable disease surveillance to identify prisoners with infectious and communicable diseases. Surveillance includes statistical record keeping, analyses of trends, and notification of reportable communicable diseases to the appropriate authorities in compliance with local and state requirements;

8. Mandate immediate medical evaluation to determine the need for isolation and quarantine for prisoners with symptoms that would suggest suspected or active untreated tuberculosis or other communicable diseases;

9. Oversee ongoing educational programs on communicable diseases for prisoners and staff that are appropriate to each audience. Programs should provide basic instruction on good personal hygiene practices, principles of disease transmission, and harm reduction. Educational programs on infection control work practices must be provided to prisoners and staff working in the following areas: laundry, housekeeping, food service, and health services;

10. Define the interaction and collaboration with local and/or state departments of public health, community health, correctional health and other agencies, and hospitals that have oversight of the health care of prisoners while they are incarcerated or when they return to the community. This collaboration includes discharge planning with linkage to community for follow-up, educational programs, surveillance and screening activities, prophylaxis, and treatment of outbreaks of communicable disease.

B. Treatment of Communicable and Infectious Diseases

Satisfactory compliance: Following the identification of prisoners with communicable diseases, institutions must provide access to appropriate treatment. Treatment of communicable diseases must follow current recommendations of CDC or other national standards-setting government bodies such as the National Institutes of Health (NIH). There must also be written policies and procedures that describe current standards of care and address other screening, identification, treatment, housing, isolation, and health education needs related to each of the communicable diseases known or suspected to be present in the prison or jail population. Examples of these diseases and the minimal requirements for compliance follow:

1. HIV infection

Principle: Due to the increase in the incarceration of individuals at high risk for HIV infection, jails and prisons must have protocols for screening and early identification as well as provide treatment for individuals with HIV infection. For many patients, HIV is a chronic disease that requires complex management with antiretroviral medications. Prisons and jail clinicians must keep current with the U.S. Department of Health and Human Services (DHHS) guidelines for the treatment of HIV. These guidelines are updated regularly, since the treatment of HIV is evolving.

Public Health Rationale: The early identification and treatment of individuals with HIV has been shown to increase survival, improve the quality of life, and offer opportunities for prevention education to prevent the further transmission of HIV within the facility and upon prisoners' release. Early intervention and treatment of women with HIV, specificly intervention during pregnancy, has been shown to decrease perinatal HIV transmission. As national treatment standards change, so must the policies and practices in jail and prison health programs to ensure that prisoners with HIV obtain the best possible outcomes.

HIV-positive prisoners should not be segregated. Quarantine undermines effective HIV education and control and wrongly suggests that HIV is casually transmitted. Since quarantine is punitive, it discourages prisoners from testing for HIV and wrongly suggests that prisoners who are not quarantined are HIV negative. As of the publication of these standards, several states require mandatory testing and segregate HIV-positive prisoners, while other states congregate HIV prisoners in specific facilities. Although it may not be appropriate to have the most complex medical services, particularly those approaching hospital level services, at every prison, clinical need, rather than HIV status, should be used for institutional assignment.

Satisfactory Compliance:

a. TREATMENT

   (1) The evolving standard of care includes a combination of anti-retroviral agents, prophylaxis for opportunistic infection, and the symptomatic treatment of conditions that occur. Jail and prison health care staff must use the current DHHS treatment guidelines in the care of prisoners with HIV.

   (2) Due to the complexity of HIV clinical management, expert clinical consultation must be available. Although HIV-positive prisoners will continue to receive primary care from prison or jail based physicians, their HIV care must be directed by clinicians with experience treating this disease. HIV specialists should supervise all HIV-related care and be available for consultation. Additional specialty and subspecialty consultation, as well as specialized diagnostic testing and treatment, should be available for HIV-positive prisoners.

   (3) To assure that primary care for HIV-positive patients is adequate, all health care providers must have current training and/or education in HIV care and management. Updated training in HIV should occur annually.

   (4) Individualized treatment plans must take into account previous antiretroviral intervention as well as a review of past and current opportunistic diseases and need for prophylaxis. The treatment plan must be discussed with the prisoner. Such a plan must address specific treatment recommendations, adherence instruction and assistance, prophylaxis and treatment of opportunistic infections, prevention and treatment of non HIV-related illnesses, risk reduction, partner notification, designated surrogacy, and referrals, if indicated, for nutritional assessment, dental care, and clinical trials.

   (5) HIV-positive pregnant prisoners must be counseled on the role of antiretroviral treatment in the prevention of perinatal transmission. These women must be offered the standard treatment for HIV-positive pregnant women as outlined in the current *NIH Guidelines for the Reduction of Perinatal Transmission.* HIV-positive pregnant women are candidates for Caesarian section.

b. SPECIAL HOUSING AND ISOLATION NEEDS

   (1) Segregation of HIV/AIDS patients is not necessary for public health purposes unless the individual is also infected with tuberculosis.

   (2) Prisoners with HIV who otherwise meet eligibility requirements for special correctional programs (e.g., work assignments, parole) must be given equal consideration.

   (3) Prisoners with HIV must be offered the same work, education, and recreational programs as uninfected prisoners.

(4) Prisoner confidentiality must be maintained in all programming and work assignments. Specific sanctions for personnel who violate medical confidentiality regarding HIV infection must be established and enforced.

c. UNIVERSAL PRECAUTIONS: Except for unusual situations when exposure to blood or body fluids is likely, correctional personnel are not required to take special precautions in managing HIV-positive prisoners. Mask, gowns, and/or gloves are not needed for performing routine duties such as feeding, escorting, or transporting HIV-positive prisoners.

d. CONTACTS: Contacts are sexual partners, needle-sharing partners, or recipients of inoculation or transfusion of HIV-contaminated blood. If identified, these individuals must receive accurate information about the infection as well as comprehensive counseling and antibody testing if desired.

e. HIV ANTIBODY SCREENING

(1) Mandatory determination of HIV antibody status is only appropriate for prospective donors of blood or other biologics.

(2) Voluntary HIV testing for the purpose of initiating HIV treatment must be available for prisoners who request it.

(3) Anyone with a clinical indication of HIV, a history of high-risk behavior, or an STD diagnosis must be encouraged to test for HIV. Testing is a component of a comprehensive clinical evaluation and a part of a voluntary counseling education program for at-risk individuals. Health care providers must receive informed consent from the prisoner-patients before counseling sessions can begin.

(4) Prison health care providers have an obligation to encourage prisoners to learn their HIV status since early treatment intervention has shown to prevent damage to the immune system, delay disease progression, and improve quality of life.

f. PREVENTION EDUCATION

(1) All prisoners must be informed of the potential for transmission of HIV infection and be advised against the sharing of needles, razors, toothbrushes, and tattooing instruments.

(2) It is the responsibility of prison and health care staff to inform prisoners about the risk of HIV infection during unprotected sexual contact and to teach prisoners safe sex practices.

(3) Peer education programs have been shown to be effective in providing HIV prevention information to prisoners. HIV education must include information about modes of transmission, prevention, treatment, and disease progression. Educational programs must also be culturally sensitive and provide scientifically accurate information as well as include the psychosocial implications of infection and the resources that are within the institution and the community.

(4) Given the potential for the spread of HIV within prisons and jails and the mortality associated with HIV, health care staff within jails and prisons must make protective barrier devices available to prisoners to reduce the spread of HIV infection.

(5) Every prisoner must be given HIV information and have access to continuing HIV education.

(*a*) Current written educational materials must be available.

(*b*) Prisoners must be offered HIV testing upon entry to the prison or jail and then offered testing every year thereafter.

(*c*) Peer HIV education for prisoners should be encouraged.

(*d*) Provisions must be made for translation of basic HIV education materials into languages spoken by prisoners. Interpreters must also be provided.

g. CONTINUING PROVIDER EDUCATION: Medical and other health care staff must have access to updated HIV information to be able to fully explain the requirements, potential benefits, and possible side effects of new treatments. These updates should be provided annually, if not more frequently.

h. CONFIDENTIALITY: Jails and prisons must develop a plan to ensure the highest degree of patient confidentiality regarding HIV status and medical condition. Staff training must emphasize the need for confidentiality and procedures must be in place to limit access to health records to only authorized individuals when it is essential to the health of the prisoners.

2. Tuberculosis

Principle: Every jail and prison must have a tuberculosis (TB) screening program. Prophylaxis and treatment should be consistent with current CDC guidelines. Once a prisoner is identified as having TB, timely and appropriate TB treatment should be initiated and the prisoner monitored to assure that treatment and follow-up care are compliant with CDC guidelines. Prisons and jails must also meet the current requirements established by the CDC for controlling TB in correctional facilities and work in partnership with public health TB control programs.

Public Health Rationale: TB prevention and treatment within prisons and jails is a major health priority because of the high rates of incarceration of individuals at risk for TB due to substance abuse, poverty, homelessness, previous incarceration, and other socio-environmental factors. In addition, persons with HIV are more likely to become infected with TB due to a depletion in the immune system. The transfer of prisoners within the jail and prison system poses an increased risk of exposure of prisoners and staff to active tuberculosis. TB can be prevented through timely and appropriate screening, prevention, and treatment of the disease.

Satisfactory Compliance:

a. SCREENING: All new admissions must be screened for TB. TB screening should include prisoners transferred from other facilities, even though they may have been previously evaluated. TB skin tests and chest radiographs are appropriate screening tools. Procedures for the use of each screening process should be based on local epidemiologic characteristics, length of stay, and the ability of the facility to conduct careful histories, physical examinations, and cross matches with regional TB registries.

b. PROPHYLAXIS AND TREATMENT

   (1) All facilities must have written policies and procedures that address prisoner refusal for testing and/or treatment for TB.

   (2) Prophylactic treatment must meet current CDC guidelines. Currently, the CDC recommends treatment for the following groups if there is no documentation of prior prophylaxis: persons with positive PPD if under 35 years old, persons with recent skin test conversions, and persons with positive PPD tests who suffer from other medical conditions that increase risk for TB (e.g., leukemia, silicosis, diabetes, end stage renal disease, immunosuppressive therapy, malnutrition).

   (3) Treatment must be based upon current CDC guidelines for the treatment of TB and for treatment of persons with HIV co-infected with TB.

   (4) All institutions must follow the current CDC guidelines for the surveillance and treatment of prisoners infected with MDR-TB, whether the disease is active or not.

   (5) Facilities must make every effort to assure timely reporting of the results to assure the most appropriate treatment intervention for the prisoner.

   (6) A directly observed therapy program must be in place to assure appropriate treatment and prophylaxis.

c. SPECIAL HOUSING AND ISOLATION NEEDS

   (1) All prisoners exhibiting symptoms of TB and those suspected of having TB must remain in single-unit medical isolation until they are no longer infectious to other prisoners and staff. The decision to remove a prisoner diagnosed with infectious TB should be made by an experienced clinician.

   (2) Negative pressure rooms must be available for the medical isolation of prisoners believed to have infectious TB. Negative pressure rooms must be tested regularly to ensure proper ventilation. If the room is being used, it must be tested daily; if it is not used, it should be tested monthly. Testing must be documented.

   (3) Patients who are bacteriologically negative, who do not cough, or who are on adequate chemotherapy need not be isolated.

d. CONTACTS

   (1) Prisoners who share cells with persons identified as having active TB or prisoners sharing air through a common ventilation system require tuberculin skin testing. If the test is negative, a repeat test must be performed 2 to 3 months later. Chest X-ray and clinical follow-up are necessary for contacts with prior positive PPD.

(2) Prisoners with active TB should be encouraged to be tested for antibodies for HIV. Information regarding the relationship between HIV and TB must be explained so that the prisoner can make an informed decision regarding HIV testing.

(3) All prisoners who might be released prior to the reading of the TB test must be provided with community referrals for follow-up care. Efforts must be made to link the prisoner with a specific treatment provider prior to discharge.

(4) All prisoners who are discharged and who are receiving anti-TB medications must be referred to the local health department or local clinical provider for follow-up care and treatment.

e. PREVENTION AND PATIENT EDUCATION

(1) Annual PPD testing for new skin reactivity, appropriate treatment, and follow-up with chest x-rays will prevent the development of active, highly communicable TB.

(2) Patients who test positive for TB must be informed that productive cough, fevers, sweats, and weight loss are danger signs that require medical consultation. The importance of covering the nose and mouth when coughing must be emphasized.

f. EMPLOYEE TESTING AND TRAINING

(1) All correctional employees must be tested for TB upon hire and again annually as a condition of employment. More frequent TB testing should be considered if TB prevalence data at the individual facility shows a need.

(2) All prison or jail staff must received TB education to help them learn the symptoms of TB and proper infection control interventions to prevent the spread of the disease within the facility.

3. **Viral hepatitis**

Principle: There must be a program to treat and prevent the spread of viral hepatitis, which is a potentially fatal communicable disease, and should include prevention education and prophylactic vaccines for hepatitis A and B. Prisons and jails must comply with CDC recommendations for prevention of viral hepatitis.

Public Health Rationale: The availability of comprehensive screening, identification, treatment, and prevention education can reduce the morbidity and mortality associated with viral hepatitis. Prison and jail health services must identify prisoners who are infected with hepatitis because it is essential that timely and appropriate immunization and, where appropriate, treatment intervention and follow-up of infected prisoners be administered. Viral hepatitis A, B, and hepatitis C in particular, are epidemic in jails and prisons. Since hepatitis infections are often sexually transmitted, it is important that facilities have prisoner prevention education programs. Furthermore, health care staff must be adequately trained by medical specialists to recognize and treat the various strains of hepatitis.

Satisfactory Compliance:

a. HEPATITIS A: Hepatitis A virus (HAV) produces a self-limited illness characterized by fever, malaise, anorexia, nausea, and abdominal discomfort followed by a jaundiced condition that usually lasts 1 to 2 weeks; however, convalescence may be prolonged. Diagnosis is established by presence of IgM antibodies to hepatitis A virus in the serum. Subsequent IgG antibodies appear at 4 to 6 weeks after onset and confer lifelong protection against reinfection. HAV is transmitted from person to person by the fecal-oral route (e.g., ingestion of food, water, or any substance that is contaminated with infected fecal material). The incubation period for hepatitis A averages 30 days.

(1) *TREATMENT OF PATIENT:* Nonspecific supportive therapy only, such as parenteral hydration if patient is anorectic and seriously dehydrated and supportive diet and medications for symptom control.

Adults with signs and symptoms of acute hepatitis should have appropriate diagnostic testing to differentiate acute hepatitis A, B, or C, and to determine if the patient has chronic hepatitis B (HBV) or hepatitis C (HCV) infection. Cases of acute viral hepatitis should be reported to the local health department.

(2) *PREVENTION:* The hepatitis A vaccine must be administered to prisoners with HIV infection, prisoners co-infected with hepatitis C, and those with chronic liver disease as well as incoming prisoners at high risk for contracting this infection. The hepatitis A vaccine should also be provided to adolescents in states where routine vaccination of adolescents is recommended. Prisoners who have a definite history of vaccination or infection with hepatitis A should not be vaccinated.

(3) *SPECIAL HOUSING, ISOLATION NEEDS, AND ENTERIC PRECAUTIONS:* Patients with hepatitis A need their own toilet during the first 2 weeks of illness and for 1 week after the onset of jaundice. Prisoners with hepatitis A must not be food handlers during this period.

(4) *IDENTIFICATION AND TREATMENT OF CONTACTS:* Cellmates, sexual contacts, other residents, and staff who have had close contact with patients must be treated prophylactically within 2 weeks of exposure to viral hepatitis with immune globulin immunization.

(5) *PREVENTION OF EPIDEMIC SPREAD AND PATIENT EDUCATION:* Feces, urine, and blood require sanitary disposal. Syringes, razors, toothbrushes, and tattooing instruments must not be misused or shared. Food handling as well as sexual contact must be avoided.

b. HEPATITIS B: Hepatitis B usually has a gradual onset with anorexia, abdominal discomfort, nausea, and vomiting. Sometimes symptoms include arthralgia and rash as well. Hepatitis B often progresses to jaundice. The mode of transmission is usually by percutaneous inoculation of blood products from an infected person (e.g., intravenous drug use, tattooing, body piercing, and acupuncture). Saliva and semen are also infectious. Exposure of mucous membranes to infective blood and sexual contact can transmit infection. The incubation period averages 60 to 120 days.

(1) *SCREENING:* Depending upon the prevalence of HBV immunity in the prison or jail population, all prisoners should either be screened for vaccination, or they should routinely receive vaccination upon admission. (See CDC's most current recommendations on hepatitis prevention and treatment in prisons and jails).

Prisoners with a history of drug use, previous jaundice, hepatitis, or transfusions must be considered at high risk for chronic hepatitis B infection and should be tested for the presence of hepatitis B surface antigen (HBSAg).

(2) *TREATMENT:* Treatment for acute hepatitis B infection is supportive. Patients with chronic hepatitis should receive a special consultation to evaluate them for treatment that is consistent with current CDC guidelines.

(3) *SPECIAL HOUSING AND ISOLATION NEEDS:* No special housing or isolation are necessary.

(4) *IDENTIFICATION AND TREATMENT OF CONTACTS:* Sexual contacts and prisoners who have shared needles, razors, toothbrushes, or tattoo instruments with patients during the previous 90 days must be offered the HBV vaccine according to CDC recommendations.

(5) *PREVENTION:* Hepatitis B is a vaccine-preventable disease. Prisoners with risk factors for HBV must be offered the vaccine, which must be administered consistent with current CDC guidelines. The vaccine provides active immunity. HBV vaccine can be used for pre-exposure and post-exposure prophylaxis.

Although a three-dose vaccine series is recommended, significant immunity can be achieve through one or two doses. Therefore, the vaccination series for hepatitis B should be initiated even if the prisoner's projected length of stay is less than 6 months. Patients who begin on the vaccination series, and who are discharged before completion of the series, should be referred for outpatient follow-up vaccination.

(6) *PATIENT EDUCATION:* HBV education must be provided to all prisoners and staff of jails, prisons, and juvenile facilities. Syringes, razors, toothbrushes, and tattooing instruments must not be misused or shared. Sexual contact must be avoided until the patient's serum is antigen-negative.

(7) *HEALTH CARE STAFF PRECAUTION:* Health care staff who come in contact with prisoners at risk for HBV or who are exposed through needle sticks with contaminated blood must be advised to take the vaccine.

c. HEPATITIS C: Hepatitis C (HCV) accounts for the majority of infections that were previously referred to as non-A, non-B hepatitis. HCV is transmitted through blood transfusions, needle sharing, sexual exposure, and occupational exposure to infected blood. A full understanding of hepatitis C is still emerging; although, substantial numbers of prisoners in states with large populations of intravenous drug users (IVDU) are infected. As of late 2001, infection rate estimates in jails and prisons ranged from 14% to 40% in certain large states. For some, chronic hepatitis C appears to be a slowly-progressive disease that may gradually advance (over 10 to 40 years) to cirrhosis. Approximately 15% of those infected with hepatitis C spontaneously clear their infection. Of those remaining 85%, only a minority will develop end stage liver disease (cirrhosis).

(1) *SCREENING:* All prisoners must be offered screening for HCV upon admission. Prisoners with a history of drug use, previous jaundice, hepatitis, or transfusions must be considered high risk and testing should be encouraged.

(2) *TREATMENT:* Treatment guidelines for hepatitis C are currently in flux. NIH guidelines recommend treatment only after liver biopsy since there is substantial toxicity associated with current treatment regimens. Hepatitis C genotypes common in the United States have been relatively refractory to interferon. However, newer combination treatments and new formulations of interferon may hold promise for patients with chronic hepatitis C infection who are at risk for developing cirrhosis. Treatment of chronic hepatitis C must be under the supervision of recognized clinical experts and be consistent with current CDC guidelines.

(3) *SPECIAL HOUSING AND ISOLATION NEEDS:* No special housing or isolation are necessary; however, health care providers must adhere to universal precautions.

(4) *IDENTIFICATION AND TREATMENT OF CONTACTS:* Sexual partners and prisoners who have shared needles, razors, toothbrushes, and tattoo instruments with patients during the previous 90 days must be clinically evaluated and monitored.

(5) *PREVENTION AND EDUCATION:* HCV education must be provided to all prisoners and staff of jails, prisons, and juvenile facilities. Because of the high prevalence of HCV in the incarcerated population, peer education and counseling are essential. Harm reduction through barriers to sexual transmission must be provided to prisoners.

4. **Sexually transmitted diseases**

   Principle: Jails and prisons must integrate screening, early identification, and treatment of individuals with sexually transmitted diseases. Rapid urine screening tests for gonorrhea and chlamydia are now available and can be effective for controlling the epidemic spread of these diseases. Treatment for STDs must be consistent with current CDC guidelines.

   Public Health Rationale: The incidence of STDs continues to increase in the population within the United States and poses a major public health problem. Within correctional facilities the increase in the incarceration of individuals at high risk for STDs is further increased by substance use and high-risk sexual behaviors. The early identification and treatment of individuals with STDs has been shown to reduce the rate of transmission to uninfected individuals and to reduce morbidity associated with these diseases. In addition, jail and prison health care staff must initiate an ongoing program of STD prevention education to prevent the further transmission of HIV infection by prisoners within the facility and upon release.

Satisfactory compliance:

a. Prisons and jails must have established relationships with local and state health departments to develop a facility plan to screen, report, and treat sexually transmitted diseases. Jail and prison health care staff must also develop data links with local health departments to ensure continuity of care and treatment for prisoners incarcerated and upon release.

b. Special consideration and treatment access must be provided for pregnant prisoners. These prisoners must be identified and treated promptly to avoid incomplete or lack of treatment prior to release.

c. All prisoners in adult and juvenile facilities must be screened for STDs upon entry.

d. Any adult or juvenile prisoners identified with an STD must be referred to an HIV program or offered HIV counseling and testing.

e. Each facility must have a written plan documenting how contact tracing will be coordinated with the local health department.

f. Treatment of STDs must follow current CDC guidelines and focus on drug regimens that minimize doses for effective treatment to reduce the likelihood of a prisoner's release prior to completion of treatment.

g. Requirements for handling common sexually transmitted diseases:

(1) SYPHILIS: Syphilis is caused by *Treponema pallidum* and characterized by a primary lesion, a secondary eruption involving skin and mucous membranes, long periods of latency, and late lesions of skin, bone, viscera, central nervous, and cardiovascular systems. Syphilis is transmitted by direct contact with moist early lesions of skin and mucous membranes and body fluids and secretions during sexual contact. Only about 10% of exposures result in infection.

(a) *TREATMENT:* Treatment protocols for syphilis are based upon the stage of the infection and are standardized by the CDC.

(b) *SPECIAL HOUSING AND ISOLATION NEEDS:* None necessary.

(c) *INVESTIGATION OF CONTACTS:* Contact tracing needs to be done according to stage of disease. Contacts require a clinical exam and a serologic test for syphilis as well as appropriate treatment and follow-up. Local health departments must be notified of all new infections.

(d) *PREVENTION AND PATIENT EDUCATION:* Patients must be taught to recognize signs of infectiousness, to avoid sexual contact, and to seek medical care if signs of infection are present.

(2) GONORRHEA: Gonorrhea is caused by *Neisseria gonorrhoeae*, which produces a purulent urethral discharge in men, a cervical and pelvic infection in women, and throat infection in both

sexes. Infection may be self-limited or progress to chronic-carrier state. Rectal infection may occur from receptive anal sex in men and women. Gonorrhea is transmitted by contact with exudates from mucous membranes of infected persons and is almost always as a result of sexual activity. Specific therapy ends communicability within hours. Incubation period is 2 to 7 days or longer.

(a) *TREATMENT:* Patients found to have diagnostic Gram stains, positive DNA probes, positive Thayer Martin cultures of discharge, or a history of recent sexual contact with an infected partner should be treated according to CDC recommendations for the specific site of infection. Patients treated for gonorrhea should also be treated for presumptive chlamydia and screened for syphilis.

(b) *SPECIAL HOUSING AND ISOLATION NEEDS:* None.

(c) *CONTACTS:* Patients may identify sexual contacts to health care providers or to trained interviewers or patients may directly inform and refer contacts for examination and treatment. State law regarding contact tracing for people in the community must be followed.

(d) *PREVENTION AND PATIENT EDUCATION:* Although antibiotics in adequate doses promptly render discharges noninfectious, patients must refrain from any sexual intercourse until post-treatment cultures are free of gonococci.

(3) GENITAL HERPES: Genital herpes is caused by herpes simplex virus types 1 and 2 (HSV-1 and HSV-2). HSV-1 is characterized by a primary infection that is usually asymptomatic. Reactivation of latent infection commonly results in herpes labialis (fever blisters or cold sores) that crust and heal in a few days. HSV-2 is predominantly associated with genital sores. HSV-1 is transmitted by direct contact with the sores or with the virus in saliva of carriers, and HSV-2 is transmitted by sexual contact. Genital herpes infection is often acquired by sexual contact with an individual who is unknowingly having an asymptomatic outbreak of herpes in the genital area. Individuals with oral herpes can transmit the virus to the genital area of a sexual partner during oral-genital sex.

(a) *TREATMENT:* Both primary infection and episodic recurrent infection must be treated according to the current CDC guidelines. The treatment reduces viral shedding and the duration of the symptoms of primary infection.

(b) *SPECIAL HOUSING AND ISOLATION NEEDS:* None; however, patients with herpetic lesions must not come in contact with immunosuppressed individuals, and health care providers must wear gloves when in contact with potentially infected lesions.

(c) *PREVENTION AND PATIENT EDUCATION:* Persons with herpes must abstain from sexual contact while the lesions are present and for 10 days after the lesions heal. Risk of transmission during symptomatic periods is unknown. However, it is advised that persons with herpes use condoms for all sexual contacts to prevent transmission. Education must be directed at minimizing transfer of infectious material and contact with sores.

(4) GENITAL WARTS: Genital warts are caused by the human papilloma virus (HPV). Most HPV infections are asymptomatic, subclinical, or unrecognized and transmitted through sexual contact that includes oral, vaginal, and anal sex. Certain serotypes of HPV are associated with the development of cervical cancer, rectal cancer, and certain head and neck cancers.

    (a) *TREATMENT:* Treatment of genital warts must be guided by the preferences of the patient and the experience of the health care provider and be based upon the current CDC recommendations.

    (b) *SPECIAL HOUSING:* None.

    (c) *CONTACTS:* Prisoners must be routinely screened for HPV during the initial intake and periodically during incarceration (at least yearly during routine primary care visit).

    (d) *PREVENTION:* All prisoners must receive education on STDs and be provided with instructions regarding the prevention of transmission through barrier methods. HIV-positive female prisoners require special diagnostic evaluation of cervical cytology to prevent rapidly progressive infection and cancer.

(5) CHLAMYDIA: Chlamydia is a bacterial infection caused by *Chlamydia trachomatis*. Most infections are asymptomatic and often go unrecognized and undiagnosed. Chlamydia is frequently associated with pelvic inflammatory disease.

    (a) *TREATMENT:* Treatment of chlamydia should be based on current CDC guidelines. As note above, presumptive treatment for gonorrhea as well as screening for syphilis is part of the treatment of chlamydial infection.

    (b) *SPECIAL HOUSING:* None.

    (c) *CONTACTS:* Female prisoners must be routinely screened for chlamydia during the initial intake and periodically during incarceration (at least yearly during routine primary care visit).

    (d) *PREVENTION:* All prisoners must receive education about STDs and be provided with instructions regarding the prevention of transmission through barrier methods.

(6) TRICHOMONAS: Trichomonas is a protozoan infection caused by *Trichomonas vaginalis*.

    (a) *TREATMENT:* Treatment of trichomonas should be based on the current CDC guidelines.

(b) *SPECIAL HOUSING:* None.

(c) *CONTACTS:* Female prisoners must be routinely screened for trichomonas during the initial intake and periodically during incarceration (at least yearly during routine primary care visit).

(d) *PREVENTION:* All prisoners must receive education on STDs and be provided with instructions regarding the prevention of transmission through barrier methods.

5. **Communicable infestations**

Principle: Prisons and jails must have procedures that prevent the onset and spread of communicable infestations.

Public Health Rationale: Infestations from dermal parasites can be prevented and controlled through proper screening and examination of prisoners upon admission and at regular intervals during their incarceration. Other factors that help in the control of infestations are proper hygiene and appropriate treatment of prisoners infested with parasites.

Satisfactory Compliance:

a. LICE: Lice infestations are caused by *Pediculus corporis* (body louse), *Pthirus pubis* (crab louse), and *Pediculus humanus capitis* (head louse). Transmission occurs from direct contact with an infested person or indirectly by contact with clothing or personal belongings. Crab lice are usually transmitted through sexual contact. Infection is communicable until the lice on the person or the person's clothing and the eggs in the person's hair and clothing have been destroyed.

   (1) *TREATMENT:* Treatment of patient must follow the current CDC recommendations.

   (2) *SPECIAL HOUSING AND ISOLATION NEEDS:* None after application of appropriate pediculocide.

   (3) *CONTACTS:* Close personal contacts must be treated if they are found to be infested.

   (4) *PREVENTION AND PATIENT EDUCATION:* Routines regarding laundering clothing and bedding (wash in hot water [55°C or 131°F] for 20 minutes or dry cleaning) to destroy nits and lice must be explained to prisoners and staff.

b. RINGWORM: Ringworm is a general term used for fungal infections of the skin, hair, and nails. Causative agents are known as dermatophytes and include: *Tenia cruris* (ringworm of groin or "jock itch"), *Tenia pedis* (ringworm of foot or "athlete's foot"), *Tenia corporis* (ringworm of body), *Tenia unguium* (ringworm of nails), *Tenia capitis* (ringworm of the scalp and beard). Ringworm infections may be transmitted through direct or indirect contact with lesions of infected persons, contaminated floors and showers, clothing, or other articles.

   (1) *TREATMENT:* Lesions may be treated with appropriate topical or oral fungicides that are consistent with current CDC recommendations.

   (2) *SPECIAL HOUSING AND ISOLATION NEEDS:* None.

(3) *PREVENTION AND PATIENT EDUCATION*

(*a*) Thorough and frequent washing of affected scalp, skin, and feet helps clear and prevent infection and recurrence. Education must include information to help patients identify lesions of ringworm and initiate or seek treatment.

(*b*) Proper laundering of towels and clothing and general cleanliness of showers, floors, and dressing room benches is necessary to prevent spread of infection. A fungicidal cleaning agent must be used for disinfection, and showers must be frequently hosed and drained.

c. SCABIES: Scabies is caused by *Sarcoptes scabiei*, a mite found in intensely itching papules or vesicles on abdomen, thighs, external genitalia, finger webs, anterior wrists, elbows, and axilla. Transmission requires intimate rather than casual skin contact. Scabies is rarely contracted from undergarments or freshly contaminated bedclothes.

(1) *TREATMENT:* Treatment aimed to eliminate the mite and treatment of complications must be consistent with current CDC guidelines.

(2) *SPECIAL HOUSING AND ISOLATION NEEDS:* None; however patients should refrain from intimate contact for 24 hours after treatment.

(3) *CONTACTS:* Educate patients and close contacts who are at risk to recognize signs of infestation and to seek treatment if signs of infestation are present.

(4) *PREVENTION AND PATIENT EDUCATION:* Launder underwear, clothing, and bedding used in prior 48 hours in hot cycles of washer and dryer.

Cross References

Health Care Facilities, II.E
Environmental Health, X

References

Infection Control

Bolyard EA, Tablan OC, Williams WW, et al. Guidelines for infection control in health care personnel, 1998. *Am J Infection Control.* 1998;26:289-354.

Centers for Disease Control and Prevention. Prevention and control of influenza: recommendations of the Advisory Committee on Immunization Practices (ACIP). *MMWR.* April 2002;51(RR-3):1-31 (or most current version).

Centers for Disease Control and Prevention. Prevention of pneumococcal diseases: recommendations of the Advisory Committee on Immunization Practices (ACIP). *MMWR.* April 1997;46(RR-8):1-31 (or most current version).

Centers for Disease Control and Prevention. Immunization of health care workers: recommendations of the Advisory Committee on Immunization Practices (ACIP) and the Hospital Infection Control Practices Advisory Committee (HICPAC). *MMWR.* December 1997;46(RR-18):1-51 (or most current version).

Centers for Disease Control and Prevention. Prevention and control of tuberculosis among patients infected with human immunodeficiency virus: principles of therapy and revised recommendations. *MMWR*. October 1998;47(RR-20):1-51 (or most current version).

Centers for Disease Control and Prevention. Prevention and control of tuberculosis in correctional facilities: recommendations of the Advisory Council for the Elimination of Tuberculosis. *MMWR*. 1996;45(RR-8):1-27 (or most current version).

Centers for Disease Control and Prevention. HIV prevention through early detection and treatment of other sexually transmitted diseases—United States: recommendations of the Advisory Council for HIV and STD Prevention. *MMWR*. July 1998;47(RR-12):1-24 (or most current version).

Centers for Disease Control and Prevention. Public Health Service Guidelines for management of health care worker exposures to HIV and recommendations for post-exposure prophylaxis. *MMWR*. May 1998;47(RR-7):1-28 (or most current version).

Centers for Disease Control and Prevention. Hospital Infections Program home page: www.cdc.gov/ncidod/hip/default.htm.

Chin J, ed. *Control of Communicable Diseases Manual*, 17th ed. Washington, DC: American Public Health Association; 2000.

Cieslak PR, Bellin E, Nadal E, et al. An outbreak of scabies in a New York City jail. *Am J Infect Control*. 1991;19:162-163.

Hammett TM. Public health/corrections collaborations: prevention and treatment of HIV/AIDS, STDs, and TB. Washington, DC: National Institute of Justice and Centers for Disease Control and Prevention. Research in brief NIJ 169590; 1998.

Johnsen C. The correctional setting. In: *APIC Curriculum for Infection Control Practice*, ed. Mosby Year Book, St. Louis, Mo; 1996.

Occupational Safety and Health Administration. Regulations: blood borne pathogens, 29 CFR 1910.1030 (2001).

Occupational Safety and Health Administration. Occupational exposure to tuberculosis proposed rule. *Federal Register,* 1997;62:54159-54309.

Parikh AI, Jay MT, Kassam D, et al. Clostridium perfringens outbreak at a juvenile detention facility linked to a Thanksgiving holiday meal. *West J Med*. 1997;166:417-419.

Tulsky JP, White MC, Dawson C, Hoynes TM, Goldenson J, Schecter G. Screening for tuberculosis in jail and clinic follow-up after release. *Am J Pub Health*. 1998;88:223-26.

Skolnick AA. Look behind bars for key to control of STDs. *JAMA*. 1998;279:97-98.

Skolnick AA. Correctional and community health care collaborations. *JAMA*. 1998;279: 98-99.

HIV

Centers for Disease Control and Prevention. HIV/AIDS education and prevention programs for adults in prisons and jails and juveniles in confinement facilities—United States, 1994. *JAMA*. 1996;275:1306-1308.

Centers for Disease Control and Prevention. HIV/AIDS education and prevention programs for adults in prisons and jails and juveniles in confinement facilities—United States, 1994. *MMWR Morb Mortal Wkly Rep*. 1996;45:268-271.

Altice FL, Mostashari F, Selwyn PA, et al. Predictors of HIV infection among newly sentenced male prisoners. *J Acquir Immune Defic Syndr Hum Retrovirol*. 1998;18:444-453.

Boudin K, Carrero I, Clark J, et al. ACE: a peer education and counseling program meets the needs of incarcerated women with HIV/AIDS issues. *J Assoc Nurses AIDS Care*. 1999;10:90-98.

Dean-Gaitor HD, Fleming PL. Epidemiology of AIDS in incarcerated persons in the United States, 1994-1996. *AIDS*. 1999;13:2429-2435.

Dubler NN, Sidel VW. On research on HIV infection and AIDS in correctional institutions. *Milbank Q*. 1989;67:171-207.

Fogel CI, Belyea M. The lives of incarcerated women: violence, substance abuse, and at risk for HIV. *J Assoc Nurses AIDS Care.* 1999;10:66-74.

Frank L. Prisons and public health: emerging issues in HIV treatment adherence. *J Assoc Nurses AIDS Care.* 1999;10:24-32.

Gostin L, Curran WJ. AIDS screening, confidentiality, and the duty to warn. *Am J Public Health.* 1987;77:361-365.

Gostin LO, Webber DW. HIV infection and AIDS in the public health and health care systems: the role of law and litigation. *JAMA.* 1998;279:1108-13.

Hankins CA, Gendron S, Handley MA, Richard C, Tung MT, O'Shaughnessy M. HIV infection among women in prison: an assessment of risk factors using a nonnominal methodology. *Am J Public Health.* 1994;84:1637-1640.

Leh SK. HIV infection in U.S. correctional systems: its effect on the community. *J Com Health Nurs.* 1999;16:53-63.

Munro D. Effective HIV/AIDS strategies, policies and programs for the correctional centre system. *P N G Med J.* 1996;39:230-233. (Prison AIDS Project, New South Wales Department of Corrective Services, Sydney, Australia.)

Smith BV, Dailard C. Female prisoners and AIDS: on the margins of public health and social justice. *AIDS Public Policy J.* 1994;9:78-85.

Tomasevski K. AIDS and prisons. *AIDS.* 1991;5 Suppl 2:S245-51.

Valerio Monge CJ. HIV/AIDS and human rights in prison. The Costa Rican experience. *Med Law.* 1998;17:197-210.

Viadro CI, Earp JA. AIDS education and incarcerated women: a neglected opportunity. *Women Health.* 1991;17:105-117.

Ward K. AIDS. HIV in prison: the importance of prevention. *Nurs Stand.* 1996;11:51-52.

Zaitzow BH. Women prisoners and HIV/AIDS. *J Assoc Nurses AIDS Care.* 1999;10:78-89.

Tuberculosis

Joint Tuberculosis Committee of the British Thoracic Society. Control and prevention of tuberculosis in the United Kingdom: Code of Practice 1994. *Thorax.* 1994; 49:1193-1200.

Kendig N. Tuberculosis control in prisons. *Int J Tuberc Lung Dis.* 1998;2:S57-63.

Levy MH, Reyes H, Coninx R. Overwhelming consumption in prisons: human rights and tuberculosis control. *Health Hum Rights.* 1999;4:166-191.

Nolan CM. Community-wide implementation of targeted testing for and treatment of latent tuberculosis infection. *Clin Infect Dis.* 1999;29:880-887.

Viral Hepatitis

Reindollar RW. Hepatitis C and the correctional population. *Am J Med.* 1999;107:100S-103S.

Sexually Transmitted Diseases

Cohen D, Scribner R, Clark J, Cory D The potential role of custody facilities in controlling sexually transmitted diseases. *Am J Public Health.* 1992;82:552-556.

Glaser JB. Sexually transmitted diseases in the incarcerated. An underexploited public health opportunity. *Sex Transm Dis.* 1998;25:308-309.

Parece MS, Herrera GA, Voigt RF, Middlekauff SL, Irwin KL. STD testing policies and practices in U.S. city and county jails. *Sex Transm Dis.* 1999;26:431-437.

Spaulding AC. The role of correctional facilities in public health: the example of sexually transmitted diseases. *Med Health R I.* 1998;81:204-206.

VI.B DRUG AND ALCOHOL DETOXIFICATION AND TREATMENT

Principle: On admission, and at any other time if indicated, prisoners must be evaluated for the presence or risk of withdrawal from alcohol, narcotics, benzodiazepines, barbiturates, and other drugs. Drug withdrawal syndromes are painful and potentially lethal. Withdrawal syndromes must be prevented, if possible, by use of appropriate pharmacologic agents and symptoms of drug withdrawal should be aggressively treated to minimize suffering. Drug treatments that emphasize harm reduction as well as rehabilitation must be an essential part of the health care program.

Public Health Rationale: Drug prohibition policies, combined with high failure rates for current abstinence treatment programs, have fueled the epidemic of mass incarceration, making the need for drug and alcohol treatment services in prisons and jails enormous. Drug withdrawal syndromes can be easily and effectively prevented or treated. Harm reduction includes successful strategies for minimizing the harmful complications of drug use and should be included in every drug treatment program.

The most commonly addictive drug used by prisoners is nicotine. Cigarette smoking is among the greatest public health dangers in our society, and prisoners should be supported in efforts to detoxify themselves from nicotine addiction.

Satisfactory Compliance:

1. Each facility must develop protocols based upon accepted national standards for the identification and management of drug withdrawal syndromes for the following drugs: nicotine, alcohol, benzodiazepine, barbiturates, cocaine, and opiates.

2. An initial medical screening and a complete medical examination must evaluate each incoming prisoner for signs or risk of drug withdrawal and drug or alcohol addiction.

3. Prisoners experiencing opiate withdrawal, or who are likely to develop opiate withdrawal, must receive a structured detoxification with methadone or other long acting opiate.

4. Prisoners enrolled in methadone maintenance treatment programs at the time of incarceration must be maintained on methadone or slowly detoxified over at least a 3 week period.

5. Prisoners at risk for alcohol, benzodiazepene, or barbiturate withdrawal must be treated with benzodiazepenes or other effective drug treatment to prevent potentially life threatening complications of these syndromes and examined at least daily by medical staff until the withdrawal syndrome is over.

6. Prisoners experiencing alcohol withdrawal must receive appropriate amounts of benzodiazepines to prevent withdrawal and to prevent delirium tremens. Severe alcohol withdrawal must be treated in an infirmary or hospital, depending on the infirmary capabilities and the severity of the withdrawal syndrome.

7. Any prisoner experiencing delirium tremens must be hospitalized for treatment of this medical emergency.

8. Prisoners addicted to barbiturates or benzodiazepenes must be treated with a tapering schedule of appropriate sedative medication to prevent serious

medical complications, including status epilepticus. The presence of complications from long term cocaine and amphetamine use must be addressed on admission.

9. Prisoners addicted to cocaine, amphetamines, or other stimulants will be evaluated for the presence of specific complications of long term use of these substances.

10. Pregnant women enrolled in methadone maintenance programs *must* be given the opportunity to continue with their regular methadone dosage until after delivery. Pregnant women addicted to opiates should be encouraged to be maintained on methadone for the duration of their pregnancy. Pregnant women addicted to opiates should be counseled about the risks of withdrawal. The decision to be maintained on methadone requires the woman's consent.

11. Prisoners who have a history of substance abuse and who desire counseling or treatment, must have programs, including counseling, available to them. Entry into such a program must be voluntary.

12. Prisoners entering smoke-free facilities, or who wish to detoxify from nicotine must be supported with smoking cessation programs as well as with nicotine-based replacement therapies (e.g., patch, gum, inhaler).

Cross References

Initial Medical Screening and Complete Medical Examination, III.A
Tobacco, VI.C
Mental Health Services, V

References

American College of Physicians, National Commission on Health Care, and the American Correctional Health Services Association. The crisis in correctional health care: the impact of the national drug control strategy on correctional health services. *Ann Intern Med.* 1992;117:71-77.

Archie CL. Obstetric management of the addicted pregnant woman. In: *Drug Dependency in Pregnancy: Managing Withdrawal.* Sacramento, Ca: Maternal and Child Health Branch, California Department of Health Services; 1992.

Center for Substance Abuse Treatment. CSAT releases guide for developing substance abuse treatment services for women in U.S. jails and prisons. *Psychiatr Serv.* 1999;50:1373.

Cohen RL. Intake evaluation in prisons and jails. In: *Clinical Practice in Correctional Medicine.* Puisis M, ed. St. Louis, Mo: Mosby Publishers; 1998.

Fogel CI, Belyea M. The lives of incarcerated women: violence, substance abuse, and at risk for HIV. *J Assoc Nurses AIDS Care.* 1999;10:66-74.

Henderson DJ. Drug abuse and incarcerated women. A research review. *J Subst Abuse Treat.* 1998;15:579-587.

Leukefeld CG, Tims FM. Directions for practice and research. In: CG Leukefeld, FM Tims, eds. *Drug Abuse Treatment in Prisons and Jails*: NIDA Research Monograph 118. Rockville, MD: National Institute on Drug Abuse; 1992.

Peters RH. Referral and screening for substance abuse treatment in jails. *J Ment Health Adm.* 1992;19:53-75.

Wexler HK. The success of therapeutic communities for substance abusers in American prisons. *J Psychoactive Drugs.* 1995;27:57-65.

Legal References

Feliciano v Gonzalez, 13 F Supp 2d 151 (DPR 1998).
Lancaster v Monroe County, 116 F3d 1419, 1425 (11th Cir 1997).
Liscio v Warren, 901 F2d 274 (2nd Cir 1990).
Pedraza v Meyer, 919 F2d 317, 318-319 (5th Cir 1990).
United States ex rel. Walker v Fayette Co., Pa., 599 F2d 573, 575-576 (3rd Cir 1979).
Palmigiano v Garrahy, 443 F Supp 956, 989 (DRI 1977).
Laaman v Helgemoe, 437 F Supp 269, 314, 314-315 (DNH 1977).
Abraham v State, 585 P2d 526, 533 (Alaska 1978).
People v Ryan, 12 Cal Rptr 2d 395, 396-397 (Cal App 1992).

VI.C TOBACCO

Principle: A comprehensive tobacco prevention and control program is an important component of a health care program for prisoners.

Public Health Rationale: Tobacco use is prevalent among prisoners. It is also the most prevalent cause of preventable morbidity and mortality in the United States, and environmental tobacco smoke exposure is a well-documented health risk to nonusers. Comprehensive public health strategies that are effective in reducing tobacco use in the community can be applied in jail and prison settings.

Satisfactory Compliance:

1. Access to tobacco products should be limited to purchase at community prices, including taxes.
2. Smoking of tobacco products should be restricted to designated areas in jails and prisons with adequate ventilation to ensure egress of the environmental tobacco smoke. Smoking must be prohibited in housing, work, education, and health care areas. Policies must be in place to ensure that there is no involuntary exposure to environmental tobacco smoke.
3. Qualified health care professionals must include screening questions about tobacco use at initial medical screening and at periodic health maintenance evaluations.
4. Health education must be provided regarding tobacco prevention and tobacco-related illnesses.
5. Prisoners must have access to effective smoking cessation programs, including nicotine replacement therapy.
6. Jail and prison staff may not use tobacco products as part of reward or incentive systems.

Cross References

Drug and Alcohol Detoxification and Treatment, VI.B
Wellness Promotion and Health Education, IX

References

Law MR, Morris JK, Wald NJ. Environmental tobacco smoke exposure and ischaemic heart disease: an evaluation of the evidence. *Br Med J.* 1997;315:973-980.

May JP, Lambert WL. Preventive health issues for individuals in jails and prisons. In: *Clinical Practice in Correctional Medicine*. Puisis M, ed. St. Louis, Mo: Mosby Publishers; 1998;259-274.

Repace JL, Jinot J, Bayard S, et al. Air nicotine and saliva cotinine as indicators of workplace passive smoking exposure and risk. *Risk Analysis*. 1998;18:71-83.

Reducing Tobacco Use: A Report of the Surgeon General. Washington, DC: US Government Printing Office; 2000.

United States Public Health Service. A Clinical Practice Guideline for Treating Tobacco Use and Dependence. *JAMA*. June 2000;283:3244-3254.

Legal References

Helling v McKinney, 113 S Ct 2475 (1993).
Webber v Crabtree, 758 F3d 460, 461 (9th Cir 1998).
Beauchamp v Sullivan, 21 F3d 789 (7th Cir 1994).
Clemmons v Bohannon, 918 F2d 858 (10th Cir 1990).

VI.D SEXUALITY

Principle: Sexual desires continue to exist for persons who are incarcerated. In addition, in some institutions, prisoners are allowed furloughs and family life visits with spouses. Regardless of institutional regulations, sexual activity occurs within adult jails and prisons and in facilities with older juveniles. Sexual activity may have significant health consequences, which must be recognized and addressed by the health service providers. The following standards are intended primarily for adult facilities, but it is incumbent on providers in facilities with younger prisoners to develop appropriate responses to sexual activity that prioritize the health and safety of the younger person.

Public Health Rationale: Sexually active men and women have special health needs associated with sexual activity that must be addressed by health care staff. Men who have sex with men and women who have sex with women while incarcerated have additional unique needs. Their health and safety depend upon availability of special health services.

Because same-gender sexual relations are banned in most institutions, all discussions with prisoners about their sexual risks or activities with other prisoners must be conducted with the utmost confidentiality. Men who have sex with men and women who have sex with women may identify themselves as heterosexual. Therefore, in an interview, a prisoner may be asked "Have you had sexual contact with men? Or with women?" Knowledge of gay lifestyles will also be of use to the health care provider in order to elicit an adequate history in a sensitive manner and to appropriately diagnose and treat associated medical conditions.

Men who have sex with men in prison or jail are at risk of being subject to sexual assault or violent attack. This is especially true for those who view themselves, or are identified by others, as homosexual. While some institutions provide special safe housing for homosexual men, such arrangements can further stigmatize their residents or result in inadequate access to programs and institutional life.

While female-to-female sexual transmission of HIV is more difficult than heterosexual transmission, it can occur. Additionally, women may have already been

exposed to sexually transmitted diseases (including HIV) by a female or male partner while outside of prison.

Autoeroticism is another sexual activity practiced by many prisoners.

Satisfactory compliance:

1. **All prisoners**
   a. Sexuality and the concomitant intimacy are inherent aspects of being
   human. From a public health point of view, all prisoners should be
   allowed to retain their identities as sexual beings and encouraged to
   develop skills for intimacy in relationships. Therefore, personal visits
   with spouses and partners, including overnight visits, should be the goal
   of correctional policy.
   b. All prisoners, including adolescents, need education and counseling
   concerning risks of sexually transmitted diseases, especially HIV, hepatitis, syphilis, and gonorrhea. Women need counseling about chlamydia, human papillomavirus (HPV), and the necessity of cervical cytology or Pap screen and may require education about contraception and
   pregnancy.
   c. Anonymous and confidential HIV antibody testing should be offered to
   all prisoners.
   d. Prisoners who are concerned about autoerotic activities should be provided with sensitive education and counseling by health care staff that
   emphasizes the normalcy of masturbation.
   e. Both men and women should be provided with condoms for HIV protection.
   f. Prisoners going on approved family visits as well as all those about to
   be released should be provided with appropriate contraception and HIV
   education.
   g. Women should be allowed to continue hormonal contraception to maintain protection for the current menstrual cycle. They should also be
   allowed to begin hormonal contraception a month before their release.
   h. Prisoners returning from furloughs and/or family visits should be provided with STD and HIV testing, if requested.

2. **Men who have sex with men**
   a. At a minimum, these men should be offered annual screening tests for:
      (1) serology for syphilis;
      (2) gonorrhea cultures—oral, urethral, and rectal;
      (3) if indicated, stool cultures for ova and parasites; and
      (4) HIV antibody test.
   b. Appropriate educational material and counseling concerning protection
   from sexually transmitted diseases, including HIV, must be provided.
   c. A basic public health role of the medical provider is to assist in the development of a violence–prevention plan that includes prevention of sexual violence, if any is revealed.

3. **Women who have sex with women**
   a. Appropriate educational material and counseling concerning protection
   from sexually transmitted diseases must be provided.

    b. A sensitive inquiry regarding current and future contraceptive needs should be provided for women who have sex with women while incarcerated. When appropriate (e.g., before release) contraceptive education, counseling, and supplies should be provided.

    c. Education should be provided regarding the fact that they are still at risk of HIV or hepatitis B transmission from an intimate partner via shared needles or other personal implements, such as frequent sharing of tooth brushes.

Cross References

Communicable Diseases, VI.A
Wellness Promotion and Health Education, IX

References

Farrow JA, Schroeder E. Sexuality education groups in juvenile detention. *Adolescence.* 1984;19:817-826.

Maeve MK. The social construction of love and sexuality in a women's prison. *ANS Adv* 1999;21:46-65.

Viadro CI, Earp JA. AIDS education and incarcerated women: a neglected opportunity. *Women Health.* 1991;17:105-117.

VI.E   DENTAL HEALTH CARE SERVICES

Principle: Comprehensive dental care must be available to all prisoners.

Public Health Rationale: Proper maintenance of the oral structures plays an important role in providing for the general well-being of prisoners.

Satisfactory Compliance:

1. An organized program of care must be available through an onsite facility or by referral.

2. Professional responsibility for the dental care program must be under the direction of a licensed dentist.

3. All necessary services required to maintain or restore the oral structures of prisoners to functional health must be available onsite or by contract with a local licensed provider.

4. There must be a program to prevent oral disease and to meet the oral hygiene needs of prisoners.

A. The Dental Health Facility

Principle: Every jail or prison institution must have a dental health facility or available route for adequate referral to an outside dental care facility.

Public Health Rationale: Dental health services must be readily accessible and are best provided through an onsite facility. Because of the particularly invasive nature of the work, the facility must meet state licensing requirements and have an infection control program that reduces the risk of infection.

Satisfactory Compliance:

1. There must be adequate resources (e.g., space, staff, funds, and equipment) to achieve program objectives.

2. A well-defined organizational structure with clear lines of authority and accountability must be established and maintained.
3. Standard operating policies and procedures must be maintained.
4. All dental personnel employed in positions that are required by state law to be licensed, registered, or certified, must be so qualified.
5. Adequate health care staff must be employed to assist in rendering efficient care. Duties may be delegated to auxiliary personnel in accordance with state law.
6. The dental health facility must be in compliance with all federal, state, and local health, safety, and infection control regulations.
7. Patients and staff must be protected from infectious and other dangerous hazards, including radiation.
8. Dental staff must be trained and equipped to handle medical emergencies.
9. In jails or prisons where dental services are contracted out, there must be an individual onsite who is designated as the dental services program coordinator.
10. There must be a formal and regular assessment of the quality of the dental services program based upon contemporary national community standards of care.
11. As a minimum, the following equipment must be available in the dental operatory:
    a. Dental spotlight, x-ray machine, and developing facilities, including panographic x-ray machine;
    b. Dental unit with hand pieces, water spray, and high-speed suction;
    c. Adjustable reclining patient chair;
    d. Operator and assistant stools; and
    e. Sterilization apparatus.

B. Dental Care

Principle: Comprehensive, preventative dental care must be provided to prisoners.

Public Health Rationale: Prevention of disease and planned care is preferable to episodic, emergency care. Services should be oriented to maintaining and restoring the oral structures of prisoners. Restoration of the dentition to satisfactory function and maintenance condition will enhance the health and well-being of prisoners.

Satisfactory Compliance:
1. Adequate records must be maintained for each patient and must contain the following: medical history, results of oral and hard and soft tissue examination, dental radiographs and interpretation, results of laboratory tests and pathology reports, diagnosis, treatment plan, reports of consultations, record of treatments and medications provided, necessary consent forms, and dental laboratory work orders.
2. The intake medical screening must include an examination of the teeth and gums. Any prisoner with emergency dental pain or problems identified at intake must be referred to a dentist promptly. Every prisoner

must have a comprehensive oral and hard and soft tissue examination performed by a dentist within 30 days of admission. The examination should include: indicated radiographs; charting of teeth including restorations, caries, missing teeth, and other pathology of the supporting structures; condition of oral mucosa and tooth-supporting tissues; oral hygiene status; occlusion; clinical exam of the major and minor salivary glands, neck for masses and lymphadenopathy, temporomandibular joints skin for color, tone, and abnormalities.

3. Follow-up services will be provided in clinically appropriate time frames as established by the dentist in conformance with national community standards for dental care. Specific follow-up appointments will be scheduled.

4. There must be a functioning recall system to ensure that prisoners are offered a dental examination, cleaning, and other prophylactic services at least every 6 months (or more frequently if indicated by clinical condition).

5. There must be an individual dental treatment plan for each patient based on an assessment and examination of the patient and that takes the length of detention into consideration.

6. All prisoners must receive appropriate instruction in oral hygiene and necessary supplies (e.g., soft toothbrushes and dental floss [or an appropriate substitute] must be available).

7. In addition to preventive services, treatment should include, at a minimum, the ability to restore the dental apparatus to adequate masticatory function as well as periodontal evaluation and therapy. Pain and infection must be resolved immediately. There must be a triage system to ensure that painful conditions are evaluated, appropriately validated, and responded to by dental or medical staff within 48 hours.

8. Treatment must be preventively oriented with the goal of maintaining the teeth and supporting structures. Teeth must not be extracted unless there are no other suitable treatment alternatives and only then under sound clinical indications.

9. Appropriate methods of pain control and anesthesia must be used. Narcotic analgesics should be available when necessary.

Cross References

Access to Care, I.B
Initial Medical Screening and Complete Medical Examination, III.A
Communicable Diseases, VI.A

References

Conte TG. Dental treatment of incarcerated individuals: for whom? how much? *J Prison Jail Health.* 1983;3:25.
Smith C. Dentists behind bars. *CDS Rev.* 1998;91:10-13,16-18.

Legal References

Harrison v Barkley, 219 F3d 132 (2nd Cir 2000).

Moore v Ernest-Jackson, 123 F3d 1082 (8th Cir 1997).
Boyd v Knox, 47 F3d 966, 969 (8th Cir 1995).
Fields v Ganer, 734 F2d at 1313, 1314 (8th Cir 1984).
Hoptowit v Ray, 682 F2d 1237 (9th Cir 1982).
Newman v State of Alabama, 503 F2d 1320 (8th Cir 1980).
Ramos v Lamm, 639 F2d 559 (10th Cir 1980) *cert. denied.* 450 US 1041 (1981).
Feliciano v Gonzalez, 13 F Supp 2d 151 (DPR 1998).
Cody v Hillard, 599 F Supp 1045 (SDSD 1984).
Williams v Scully, 552 F Supp 431 (SD NY 1982).
Williams v Director of Health Services, 542 F Supp 883 (SD NY 1982).
Rue v Estelle, 503 F Supp 1265, 1312-13 (SD Tex 1980).
Laaman v Helgemoe, 437 F Supp 956 (DNH 1977).
Battle v Anderson, 376 F Supp 402 (ED Okla 1974).

VI.F   EYE AND VISION SERVICES

A.   Eye and Vision Care

Principle: Eye and vision care services, including the diagnosis, treatment and visual rehabilitation of ocular and visual disorders and diseases, must be available to all prisoners.

Public Health Rationale: Eye and vision disorders affect a prisoner's ability to work, to learn, and to pursue leisure activities. Prevention, early diagnosis, treatment, and rehabilitation of eye disorders, diseases, and injuries can prevent long-term visual impairment and blindness. As the prison population ages and increases in number, more prisoners will develop acute and chronic ocular and visual conditions that are amenable to treatment.

Satisfactory Compliance:

1. A vision care program that includes screening must be supervised by an ophthalmologist or optometrist and conducted consistent with national community standards of care promoted by the American Academy of Ophthalmology and the American Optometric Association.

2. All prisoners must have a vision screening within 30 days of entrance into the correctional system and every 1 to 2 years thereafter consistent with the ocular and visual condition of the prisoner. There must be earlier screening for prisoners whose vision interferes with the activities of daily living. A trained nurse, optometrist, or trained independent licensed provider should perform the screening and refer all prisoners who fail the screening for a vision examination by an optometrist or ophthalmologist. The screening should include eye health, refractive status, and binocular function. All prisoners over 40 years of age should be seen by an ophthalmologist or optometrist within 30 days of admission for a glaucoma evaluation and any other visual care deemed necessary by the examining provider.

3. All patients who fail the initial screening should be provided with a comprehensive vision examination by an ophthalmologist or optometrist. Prisoners requiring more specialized care should be referred for specialty consultation.

4. Appropriate ophthalmic eyewear must be provided to all prisoners who require it. Eyewear should be provided within 4 weeks of a diagnosed need.

Those prisoners whose visual or ocular impairment is painful, sight threatening, and/or life vulnerable, must be provided with necessary treatment (e.g., medication, corrective eyewear on an emergency basis) and should be housed in the infirmary or other protected area pending receipt of appropriate treatment. Prisoners who require corrective eyewear must be provided with the equipment at no cost.

5. All eyewear (e.g., frames, lenses, occupational eyewear, and contact lenses) must conform to the most recent American National Standards Institute (ANSI) Z 80.1 and Z 87.1 standards.

6. Adequate clinical facilities, personnel, and equipment must be accessible or located within the health facility. Where specialist examinations are performed within the facility, the equipment available should be acceptable according to contemporary national standards of community care.

7. All results from screening and examination should be confidential and maintained in the prisoner's health care record.

B. Eyewear

Principle: All prisoners must be provided with appropriate eyewear for their special visual needs for education and training, work, and leisure activities.

Public Health Rationale: Prisoners need proper eyewear and eye protective devices to maximize vision and prevent occupational injury and illness.

Satisfactory Compliance:

1. Occupational areas must should conform to OSHA standards (currently Title 29, Part 19101.33) that identify eye-hazardous work areas and require the wearing of appropriate eye protection. Work areas not covered by these standards must be evaluated by an ophthalmologist or optometrist who will identify eye-hazardous areas and prescribe appropriate eye protection devices for prisoner workers. Other preventive measures may also be required.

2. Prisoners' eye and visual examination record must be screened upon job assignment to evaluate whether or not the prisoner has the necessary visual function for the tasks required.

Cross References

Specialty Consultative Services, III.D
Children and Adolescents, VII.B

References

Cahill JI, Woolsey T. United States Department of Health, Education, and Welfare, the National Eye Institute: Summary and critique of available data on the prevalence and economic and social costs of visual disorders and disabilities. Bethesda, MD: DHEW;1976:1-24.

American National Standard Practice for Occupatonal and Educational Eye and Face Protection. New York, NY: American National Standards Institute;1979:21-24.

Requirements for First Quality Prescription Ophthalmic Lenses. New York, NY: American National Standards Institute; 1972.

Counseling and Accreditation Program of the Council on Clinical Optometric Care. St. Louis, Mo: American Optometric Association; 1984.

Boccumni, P. *The Screening and Treatment Program for Vision and Learning Disabilities among Juvenile Offenders*. San Bernardino, Calif: Clinical Services Division, County of San Bernardino Probation Department; 1984.

Bachara GH, Zaba JN. Learning disabilities and juvenile delinquency. *J Learning Disabilities*. 1978;11:58-62.

Blew, CH, McGillis D, Bryant G. Project New Pride; An Exemplary Project. National Institute of Law Enforcement and Criminal Justice, Law Enforcement Assistance Administration. Washington, DC: US Department of Justice; 1977:41.

Occupational Safety and Health Standards. Subpart 1, Personal Protective Equipment. Code of Federal Regulations, Title 29, Chapter XVII, Part 19101.33.

Legal References

Koehl v Dalsheim, 85 F3d 87 (2nd Cir 1996).

Devivo v Butler, 1998 US Dist LEXIS 17719 (SD NY 1998).

VI.G PHARMACY SERVICES

Principle: Every jail and prison must have a pharmacy appropriate to the size of the prisoner population served.

Public Health Rationale: Pharmaceuticals are essential to the treatment and control of many acute and chronic illnesses and are an integral component of any health care program. It is only through an appropriately staffed and equipped pharmacy that medications can be provided to patients who need them. Having a functioning pharmacy will allow medications to be administered in a timely manner and according to physician orders. Doses and dose schedules must conform to current national standards of community care. A well-administered pharmacy will help improve clinical outcome. It is also important that the correctional pharmacy be able to handle prompt identification and replacement of medications that are confiscated.

Satisfactory Compliance:

1. Each jail or prison must designate a secure area for the storage of all medications. Pharmacy activities and pharmaceutical storage must be in an area physically separate from other activities. The pharmacy must comply with state pharmacy regulations that apply to community-based pharmacies.

2. Every institution must have access to the professional services of a licensed pharmacist who will provide regular and general supervision of pharmacy activities. The pharmacist will approve all pharmacy activities and assure that they conform to state regulations. The pharmacist must prepare regular reports for the medical staff summarizing drug inventory and patterns of over-the-counter and prescription drug use at the institution. Only a pharmacist or properly licensed and supervised technician as provided for by the applicable state law can dispense medication.

3. Nonprescription medications may be made available in the correctional institution at places other than the health services facility such as the commissary after consultation with the medical staff. Specific rules governing the dispensing of these medications must be written.

4. All other medication must be administered only by trained health care staff as permitted by local or state law. The administration of each dose of med-

ication must be documented for inclusion in the medical record. Medications not administered must be accounted for and returned to the pharmacy daily.

5. In facilities with formularies, there must be a mechanism for ordering and promptly securing non-formulary items.

6. In facilities in which health services staffing is not sufficient to administer all medication doses, distribution must be done by specially trained correctional staff in sealed single doses packaged by appropriate pharmacy staff and labeled with patient's name and medication name, dose, and directions.

7. If multiple doses of medications are dispensed to patients, they must be in containers clearly labeled with the patient's name and medication name, dose, and directions.

8. Liquid forms of psychiatric medications must be available. Attempts should be made to make these liquid medications palatable.

9. Medication must only be prescribed by appropriately trained, legally authorized personnel on schedules consistent with currently accepted national community standards of clinical practice and pharmaceutical science.

10. Medication must be prescribed only after a patient evaluation that should include a medical history, physical exam, assessment, and diagnosis.

11. Narcotics and other controlled substances and drugs that are dangerous or toxic or those subject to abuse by prisoners must be administered under well-controlled conditions and their ingestion by the patient observed by the staff.

12. Written and verbal education about the use and effects of medications must be available for prisoners.

13. Emergency supplies of life-sustaining drugs must be maintained onsite.

14. Expired or unused medications must be transferred or disposed of in an appropriate manner that is consistent with federal, state, and local laws.

Cross Reference

Health Care Facilities, II.E

Legal References

Johnson v Hay, 931 F2d 456 (8th Cir 1991).
Spellman v Edwards, 715 F2d 269 (7th Cir 1983).
Newman v Alabama. 349 F Supp 278 (5th Cir 1978).
Williams v Edwards, 547 F2d 1206 (5th Cir 1977).
Nelson v Prison Health Services, 991 F Supp 1452 (MD Fl 1997).
Feliciano v Gonzalez, 13 F Supp 2d 151 (DPR 1995).
Madrid v Gomez, 889 F Supp 1146, 1258 (ND Ca 1995).
Cody v Hillard, 599 F Supp 1025 (SDSD 1984).
Lightfoot v Walker 486 F Supp 504 (SD Ill 1980).
Ruiz v Estelle, 503 F Supp 1025 (SD Tex 1980).
Goldsby v Carnes, 365 F Supp 395 (WD Mo 1973) (consent decree), *modified*, 429 F Supp 370 (WD Mo 1973).

VI.H   DISTANCE-BASED MEDICINE

Principle: Distance-based medicine should supplement, but not replace, access to medical care providers and specialists.

Public Health Rationale: Distance-based medicine (also referred to as telemedicine) is the use of telecommunications techniques to provide or support clinical care. It includes delivery and provision of health care and consultative services and transmission of information related to care. It may also incorporate direct clinical preventive, diagnostic, and therapeutic services; consultative and follow-up services; remote monitoring, including remote reading and interpretation of results of patient's procedures; rehabilitative services; and patient education provided in the context of delivering health care to individuals.

While distance-based medicine can provide medical expertise to remote areas, reduce professional isolation, and lower travel costs, it can also restrict the amount and quality of personal interaction between a patient and his or her health care provider. The quality of medical care may also suffer when the distant consultant is unaware of local services, both in or near the jail or prison, when the distant consultants lack direct knowledge of the patient's condition, or when emergencies occur after a consultation and the specialist is unavailable for direct examination of the patient. In addition, factors such as imperfect transmission quality, the lack of hands-on diagnosis, and the further isolation of prisoners from independent medical institutions, should all be weighed in decisions to use distance-based medicine for diagnosis and treatment. Telemedicine's availability can become an excuse to ignore multiple impediments to access to quality care equivalent of that provided in the outside community.

Satisfactory Compliance: The use of distance-based medicine in a correctional context must provide the following minimums:

1. Clear policies outlining the circumstances under which the facility will allow individuals to be treated through distance-based medicine techniques. Such policies must include:
   a. Arrangements for "hands on" evaluations and treatments when the requirements of the physical examination exceed the capabilities of the remote-site personnel or the equipment.
   b. A mechanism through which patients can be seen by appropriately trained health care providers when necessary.
   c. Written minimum equipment standards, including transmission speed, resolution, and audio quality.
   d. Presence of an onsite health care provider when the patient is being seen at a distance by a specialist.
2. Patient consent, documentation, and storage of information
   a. Patients must consent to a distance-based medicine consultation, just as they do to in-person medical consultation;
   b. Distance-based practitioners must provide a note documenting the encounter. This note must conform to the standards in the Health Care Records section of these standards.
   c. If images will be recorded as part of the diagnostic or therapeutic process, consent forms should include discussion of the capture and use of images.

These materials (images) are part of the health care record and must be handled with the same protections for confidentiality and kept for the same amount of time as other parts of the record.

d. Telemedicine consultation with prisoners must not be used for training purposes, and prisoners must not be asked to consent to their use for educational or research purposes.

3. *Quality improvement:* The use of distance-based medicine must be monitored in the quality improvement process. Such monitoring must include quality of care aspects.

Cross References

Quality Improvement, II.B
Specialty Consultative Services, III.D

References

Bonnin A. Medical tele-imaging: a good chance for the future. *Bull Acad Natl Med.* 1999;183:1123-1136.
Fletcher DM. Telemedicine technology in correctional facilities. *J AHIMA.* 1998;69:68-71.
National Commission on Correctional Health Care. Position statement on the use of telemedicine technology in correctional facilities. *J Corr Health Care.* 1998;5:1.

VI.I FOOD SERVICES AND NUTRITION

Principle: Food should be wholesome, safe for human consumption, nutritionally adequate, and prepared and served in a sanitary manner and environment.

Public Health Rationale: Adequate diets that meet nationally recognized standards are an essential element of general well-being. There are a number of medical conditions that require special diets to promote health.

Foodborne disease, whether from intoxication or infection, is an ongoing public health concern. Food may serve as a medium for the growth of bacteria and other microorganisms and for the production of bacterial growth and the proliferation of bacterial toxins. Food may also serve as a vehicle for the transmission of chemical toxins or poisons.

Satisfactory Compliance:

1. The regular diet served in jails and prisons must meet the minimum standards established by the National Research Council for calories, vitamin, mineral, fat, protein, and carbohydrate content with respect to the age, gender, and health status of the prisoners. The diet must also be appetizing and include the daily recommended variety of foods such as fresh and raw fruits and vegetables.

2. Menu planning and implementation must be supervised by a registered dietician.

3. The regular diet or prescribed therapeutic diet must be provided to prisoners in segregation. Food should not be used for punishment or discipline.

4. There must be policies and procedures that allow health care staff to order therapeutic diets for prisoners whose medical conditions require modifications to the regular diet. Therapeutic diets must meet national standards

established by such groups as the American Dietetic Association. The diets must be appetizing and include the same variety of foods as the regular diets, except to the extent that they are prohibited for medical reasons. The preparation of menus and meals must be supervised by a registered dietician.

5. Housing should not be determined by special dietary needs.
6. When vegetarian or religious diets are provided they must be nutritionally adequate and appealing.
7. Food service operations and equipment must comply with the recommended standards of the current Food and Drug Administration (FDA) Food Code or appropriate state or local regulations and national standards such as the National Sanitation Foundation. Food service inspections must be conducted on a quarterly basis by a local, state, or federal food service inspecting agency or by a qualified institutional staff member who does not work directly for the food services program and who has knowledge of food sanitation practices. Records of such inspections, documenting level of compliance with standards of the referenced manual or equivalent state regulations, must be maintained. Staff-conducted quarterly inspections and annual inspections by appropriate external agencies should be scheduled and done to monitor the program.
8. In addition to complying with federal, state, and local health and sanitation standards, including standards in the FDA Food Code, jails and prisons must make sure that prisoners who work in the food preparation or service areas are trained, that there are policies and procedures regarding and enforcing proper hand washing, and that each facility develops and implements a Hazard Analysis Critical Control Point (HACCP) plan. In particular, the food service operation must:
   a. Provide food storage facilities to ensure proper refrigeration and preservation of all foods to prevent foodborne illnesses and food wastage.
   b. Practice sanitary and safe food handling at all times. Continual training in sanitary and safe food handling should be provided to all staff and prisoners who work as food handlers.
   c. Provide food preparation and service areas adequate for the number of people to be served. Food preparation and service areas should be equipped in accordance with basic food practices for food preparation and service.
   d. Provide dry storage facilities with proper temperature, ventilation, vermin protection, and cleanliness for the storage of nonperishable foods.
   e. Provide dining room(s) of adequate size to meet the needs of the number of people to be served. Dining rooms should be well lighted and ventilated.
   f. Provide clean uniforms to be worn at all times that will be machine washed by the facility.
   g. Maintain all areas and equipment for food preparation, storage, and service in a clean and sanitary condition.

Cross References

Quality Improvement, II.B
Environmental Health, X

Legal References

Burgin v Nix, 899 F2d 733, 734 (8th Cir 1990).

French v Owens, 777 F2d 1250, 1255 (7th Cir 1985), *cert. denied*, 479 US 817, 107 S Ct 77 (1986).

Campbell v Canthron, 623 F2d 503, 508-509 (8th Cir 1980).

Pritchett v Page, 2000 US Dist LEXIS 11559 at 14-18.

Gordon v Sheahan, 1997 WL 136699, 1997 US Dist LEXIS 16823 (ED Pa).

Talley v Amarker, 1996 WL 660930, 1996 US Dist LEXIS 16823 (ND Ill).

Dye v Sheahan, 1995 WL 109318, 1995 US Dist LEXIS 3027 (ND Ill).

VI.J   PALLIATIVE CARE, PAIN, AND SYMPTOM MANAGEMENT

Principle: The health care staff of each jail and prison must provide a patient-centered palliative care program for the effective response to physical discomfort, including timely and ongoing interventions for symptom control and pain management. Palliative care services must be available in the infirmary and all housing areas and prisoners must have access to outside specialty consultation when indicated.

Public Health Rationale: Prisoners often have a variety of health problems, including chronic, progressive, debilitating, and degenerative conditions as well as acute illnesses. In addition to curative treatment, these patients need symptom control, pain management, and interventions to maintain or restore function. For this reason, both palliative and acute care are appropriate aspects of a total health care plan. At the onset of illness, curative care will predominate but, as cure becomes less likely and the patient nears death, palliative care will increasingly govern the care goals and treatment regimen.

The under-treatment of pain is a widespread phenomenon that is especially evident in the correctional setting, particularly when prisoners have a history of prior drug abuse. There is a risk of overlooking or undervaluing the pain of patients with prior histories of drug use. Increasing pain is characteristic of progressive chronic disease and complaints of pain *must* be evaluated and *must not be dismissed* as evidence of malingering or drug-seeking behavior. Patients with certain conditions, including HIV/AIDS, benefit significantly from pain care administered by pain specialists.

Jails and prisons contain physical barriers, require security restrictions, and impose bureaucratic regulations that may exacerbate patient symptoms and impede the provision of palliative care. Temperature changes, dust, long corridors with stairs that obstruct mobility; diets that do not provide nutritional variation or supplements; and inflexible rest, exercise, mealtime and visiting schedules may fail to accommodate the therapeutic needs of patients and may hinder patients' ability to manage their activities of daily living (ADLs). Certain conditions, including HIV/AIDS, arthritis, cancer, congestive heart failure, and chronic obstructive pulmonary disease may be far harder to manage in jails and prisons than in the community. Health care staff should be advocates for a comprehensive palliative care program as a standard component of all chronic care management.

Satisfactory compliance:

1. It is the responsibility of the health care team to assess each chronically ill inmate for acute, palliative, and restorative care needs; to seek expert advice

when necessary; and to coordinate all parts of the care plan. The team must document its assessments and coordinate with correctional staff to ensure that the plan recognizes the imperatives of correctional practice and humane prisoner treatment.

2. Standing treatment protocols and clinical guidelines must address the palliative care needs of chronically and acutely ill patients. Palliative protocols and individual patient care plans must anticipate both routine and crisis care and address issues including, but not limited to, pain, fatigue, anxiety, depression, sleep disturbances, nausea, diarrhea, shortness of breath, and inability to manage ADLs. Some palliative care plans will require the involvement of mental health staff and may include use of psychotropic medications. Individualized care plans must be documented in prisoners' health records.

3. If patients are to provide truly informed consent to palliative care, they also must be assured of continued access to curative care. Medical prognosis combined with prisoner wishes and values will determine the relative balance of curative and palliative interventions. Palliative care should be an adjunct to curative care plans.

4. There should be a unified health record for each prisoner that contains plans for acute, palliative, and mental health care.

5. All health care providers must be trained in basic palliative care theory and techniques and consultation on symptom management should be available, as needed, from palliative care experts.

6. The facility-based medical director is responsible for assessing how specific security measures may affect a patient's medical treatment plan and for negotiating the elements of that plan with correctional officials. Security should be consulted about the implementation of treatment plans that require varying prison routine in ways that may affect security arrangements. Correctional staff should be involved in crafting procedures that facilitate palliative care, but not in making individual patient care decisions. The correctional administration should be engaged in planning policies and procedures that could permit extra showers, access to special meals, possession of durable medical equipment, modification of visiting, and other variations that institutional rules would normally prohibit.

7. If correctional staff are involved in discussions about patient care, all efforts must be made to protect prisoner privacy and confidentiality. For this reason, corrections officers must receive special training in safeguarding medical information and must be impressed with the need to respect patient confidentiality. Correctional institutions may require security staff to sign agreements regarding the protection of confidential medical information. Security staff may not have access to medical records and any disclosure of health care information can take place only with the prisoner's prior knowledge and agreement. Patient information must be discussed with security personnel only on a need-to-know basis and be limited to information necessary to accommodate institutional regulations to meet patient care needs.

8. Palliative care must be available in all jails and prisons and not restricted to particular residential settings since limited availability of palliative care

may force prisoners to choose between effective medical care and other programs or services. The health care system in each jail or prison must be able to deliver palliative care in all medical and residential settings and not be limited to the infirmary or to particular housing sections. The fact that a prisoner is receiving palliative care must not deprive him or her of other institutional resources. Reasonable accommodation is necessary to allow patients to participate in programs and receive services.

9. When specialized services are not available within a facility, prisoners must have timely access to outside resources and should not be subjected to lengthy or painful transport procedures. Some clustering may be advantageous both for inmates and for administrators for patients who need frequent access to specialty care. In particular, some patients with HIV/AIDS and those co-infected with other diseases may benefit if transferred to facilities near major medical centers where specialty consultation and care are readily available and accessible.

10. The central issue in palliative care is the effective management of pain, which must be provided for patients who need it, including those who abused drugs prior to incarceration. Complaints of pain should be assessed in light of the patient's diagnosis, prognosis, and current analgesia regimen. Consultation with pain specialists may be necessary, but should not delay treatment. Because medications used to treat certain illnesses, such as HIV/AIDS, may reduce the efficacy of analgesia and lead to withdrawal, dosages should be adjusted as indicated. Acupuncture, relaxation techniques, and other nontraditional pain management interventions *with demonstrated efficacy* should also be considered.

Cross References

Chronic Care Management, IV
Information Systems, II.A

References

Anno BJ, Dubler NN. Ethical consideration and the interface with custody. In: Anno BJ. *Correctional Health Care: Guidelines for the Management of an Adequate Delivery System—2001 edition.* Washington, DC: National Institute of Corrections; in press.
Dubler NN. The collision of confinement and care: end-of-life care in prisons and jails. *J Law Med Ethics.* 1998;26:149-156.
Post LP, Dubler NN. Palliative care: a bioethical definition, principles, and clinical guidelines. *Bioethics Forum.* 1997;13:17-24.
Meier D, et al. Improving palliative care. *Ann Intern Med.* 1997;127:225-230.

VI.K   HOSPICE CARE

Principle: Prisoners at the end of life should be provided with a range of hospice services, including flexible rules for visits by family and close friends, spiritual counseling, and management of pain and other symptoms. Patients should be able to die in a supportive environment, in dignity, without pain and, whenever possible, in the company of family and friends, including other prisoners.

Public Health Rationale: Jails or prisons that care for prisoners at the end of life must meet the needs of patients, families, and friends who are engaged in anticipatory grieving as they face the reality of impending death. Because family participation is central to hospice care, correctional institutions should develop hospice programs as close as possible to those localities where prisoners' families live. When appropriate, correctional administration and health care staff must also advocate for compassionate release (called "reduction in sentence" in the federal system) for prisoners who no longer pose a threat to public safety.

Satisfactory Compliance:

1. Every correctional system must have an effective process for consideration of and advocacy for compassionate release for dying prisoners. Because terminal conditions may deteriorate rapidly, review and decision about compassionate release should be conducted in a timely and efficient manner and should not preclude enrollment in a hospice program. The principal correctional medical authority should advocate, whenever feasible and appropriate, for compassionate release from custody and referral to community medical and hospice programs.

2. Whenever a chronically or terminally ill inmate is about to be released, whether through compassionate release, by parole, or at the conclusion of his or her sentence, the health care staff must develop a discharge plan that is designed to assure continuity of care after release by access to medication, community resources, and other support. This plan must be documented in the patient's health record.

3. When compassionate release is not possible, terminally ill patients must be offered hospice services that are provided jointly by prison health and community programs, if possible, and governed by the community standard. The responsible medical authority should establish formal arrangements with community hospice programs to ensure expert consultation and other services.

4. Before a prisoner is designated medically appropriate for hospice services, a physician who has not previously been involved in the case as a primary provider must review the medical record, examine the patient, and determine that the patient is dying because of medical conditions that are not reversible. This assessment should focus on the prisoner's condition, likely prognosis, treatment history, and the available therapeutic options. The review should determine whether the patient can benefit from aggressive cure-oriented treatment or whether the patient is dying and should be in a hospice program that emphasizes comfort measures. No patient should be placed in a hospice program for administrative or medical convenience or when reasonable therapeutic options remain available.

5. Enrollment in a hospice program must be a capacitated patient's choice. If the patient is incapacitated, the family, friends, or other surrogate deciding for the patient must evaluate and consent to or refuse hospice care at the end of life.

6. Hospice care constitutes a subset of palliative care and, in the United States, the term "hospice" refers to a specific, programmatic model for delivering

palliative care. Aspects of palliative care (e.g., pain management) are appropriate even at the early stages of debilitating illness; however, palliation typically becomes the predominant emphasis as illness advances and cure becomes less likely. In contrast to palliative care, which should be integrated into the regular institutional health care structure, hospice care should be provided in a specialized unit with trained staff. If no hospice program exists in a correctional institution, hospice services should be provided in the infirmary to avoid relocating the patient at the end of life, severing relationships with other prisoners, and increasing the isolation, loneliness and fear that often accompany dying. If a prisoner wishes to move to a formal hospice program, that option should be available within the correctional system and such request should receive timely consideration.

7. Like palliative care, hospice care must accommodate institutional concerns about safety and security. Models for adjustments in facility rules to meet the medical and emotional needs of the patient and family should be negotiated by health care and security staff. Working collaboratively, this interdisciplinary team should develop end-of-life care plans that do not compromise institutional security.

8. Every hospice program should have sufficient health care staff to provide all necessary services to the entire hospice population. Skilled care providers must be responsible for the development, implementation, and monitoring of all care plans.

9. The judicious use of prisoner volunteers in the correctional hospice program can benefit both patients and volunteers by providing opportunities for supportive and consistent relationships. Selected prisoner volunteers may be engaged only to supplement professional staff by performing specified nonprofessional tasks with the consent of the patient. Use of appropriately screened and trained prisoners may be encouraged, but must never substitute for professional care staff. For this reason, no prisoner who is or was a professional health care provider or has prior health care training must ever be used in a health care providing role. Prisoners who apply to work in hospice must be screened for emotional and intellectual ability and trained in specially designed programs. Volunteers' tasks should be limited to engaging the patient in conversation; acting as a 'buddy' to someone without family; non-strenuous recreational activity; and, in selected cases, feeding, assistance with dressing, and transportation by wheelchair. Prisoners must not assist with bathing, toileting, wound care, lifting, or other 'hands-on' activities that might be considered intimate or compromising to the patient's dignity. Prisoner assistants should never be permitted to engage in tasks that require professional skill or judgment, such as taking vital signs or giving medication, or activities that expose them to patient information, such as reviewing the medical chart or scheduling examinations. All care and the activities of volunteers should be supervised by a licensed health care provider and all care should ultimately be the responsibility of professional medical staff.

10. Special visiting rules should be established for family (defined not only in terms of the traditional family but also as "those to whom the death of the

prisoner matters"). When there is no family involved, and other prisoners function as family, special accommodations should be considered to permit these prisoners to support the hospice patient in the dying process. The hospice staff should facilitate contact between dying patients and family or friends from whom they have become estranged.

11. Prisoners in hospice programs or receiving hospice care in the infirmary may require substantial medication, including narcotics, at the end of life to control pain and suffering. Rather than shortening life, these medications may actually be life-prolonging and should always be considered as an appropriate part of end-of-life care. Because the prescription and delivery of medication take place in the correctional setting, both therapeutic and security concerns should be considered in developing a system that provides effective drug therapy while protecting against possible abuse. Physicians should prescribe the medication the patient needs and, when indicated, medication should not be limited to standard formulary items. Existing medical delivery systems should be modified to make narcotic medications readily available within the medical unit. When prisoners who are in hospice programs are discharged into the community through compassionate release, parole, or completion of sentence, they should be provided with medication for at least 2 weeks or until they may reasonably be expected to obtain necessary community-based follow-up care.

12. Palliative care and hospice services should respond to issues of language, culture, religion, and relationships with family, friends, and other prisoners. Accommodations in prison routine, such as adjusted visiting hours, modified diets, and religious ceremonies, can assist patients, families, staff, and other prisoners in their adjustment to dying and acceptance of death. The correctional administration and the medical and hospice staff should consider creating rituals and ceremonies to mark the death of an inmate and to permit staff, family, and other prisoners to mourn together. Critical incident debriefing and stress reduction resources for staff and volunteers should be part of the hospice program.

Cross Reference

Palliative Care, Pain, and Symptom Management, VI.J

References

Fox E, Landrum-McNiff K, Zhong Z, Dawson NV, Wu AW, Lynn J, for the SUPPORT Investigators. Evaluation of prognostic criteria for determining hospice eligibility in patients with advance lung, heart or liver disease. *JAMA.* 1999;282:1638-1645.

Maull FW. Issues in prison hospice: toward a model for the delivery of hospice care in a correctional setting. *Hospice J.* 1998;13:57-82.

Ratcliff M, Cohn F. Hospice with grace: reforming care for terminally ill inmates. *CT Feature.* 1999.

Russell MP. Too little, too late, too slow: compassionate release of terminally ill prisoners—is the care worse than the disease? *Weidener J Public Law.* Spring 1994:799-817.

VI.L   END-OF-LIFE DECISION MAKING

Principle: Prisoners approaching the end of life face many of the same profound issues as other dying patients and, although their range of choices may be constrained by their confinement, have rights of self-determination that should not be unnecessarily abridged. Protocols should ensure that patient decisions are voluntary, uncoerced, and based on medical information that is complete and comprehensible. Particular attention must be paid to protecting the patient's choices to reject life-sustaining treatment, if desired, and not to have the dying process prolonged.

Public Health Rationale: Jails and prisons are places where liberty is constrained and individual independent decision making fettered. It is often impossible to distinguish between a refusal of care and a denial of care. Decisions to permit or accept death implicate concerns about the prisoner-patient's autonomy, the accuracy of information that has been provided about diagnosis, prognosis and therapeutic options, and the quality of the acute and comfort care that has been delivered. While patients dying in the community are frequently concerned about receiving unwanted life-sustaining interventions, prisoners at the end of life risk being deprived of treatment they require. To protect prisoners from possible coercion, their right to make authentic decisions must be supported by processes that involve independent persons empowered to make independent inquiries and evaluations of the decision-making process.

Satisfactory compliance:
1. Advance directives, including health care proxy appointments and living wills, must be available to chronically and acutely ill prisoners. Advance directives must be presented as a standard part of chronic and acute care for prisoners who choose to address prospective health care decisions.
2. Prisoners must be encouraged to consider advance directives when they are still decisionally capable—before the effects of illness or disease have reduced their ability to consider the benefits, burdens, and risks of alternative future treatment options. Before executing an advance directive, the prisoner must be informed about the diagnosis, prognosis, and care options both in the facility and in other institutions in the system; the consequences of creating an advance directive; and the availability of palliative and hospice care services. A prison chaplain, community clergy, or prisoners' rights advocate should be available to talk with prisoners about their treatment planning options. Advanced directives must be made a permanent part of the patient's health record.
3. The correctional setting does not always promote the exercise of patient autonomy or the honoring of patient wishes. Because the voice of the patient is the one that must be enhanced and respected, the living will should be encouraged as the preferred advance directive and used as the first line of information about health care wishes at the end of life.
4. Health care proxy appointments (encouraged in the community) risk setting up conflicts of authority in a correctional institution. Because of this possibility, they are less favored than living wills, which explicitly state prisoners' actual preferences. Prisoners should be permitted to appoint the

family members or friends who know them best, understand their values and preferences, and are willing to accept the responsibility for end-of-life decision-making as their health care proxies. When a prisoner has no close family or friends, a chaplain in the correctional institution (preferably one at a community facility) may be chosen to act as health care proxy. Health staff at the facility should not serve as proxies. It is not advisable for a prisoner to serve as a health care proxy unless he or she is a member of the patient's immediate family.

5. Linguistic and cultural barriers to communication must be addressed before a discussion about advance directives can be legally and ethically adequate. Advance directives in the correctional facility should be modeled on those adopted by the state in which the facility is located. In the federal system, advance directives may be modeled after the forms used by the Veterans Health Administration, which are drafted to meet federal requirements.

6. Do-not-resuscitate (DNR) orders may be appropriate at the end of life. It is especially important that they be available so that a patient is not needlessly burdened with resuscitation and intubation. DNR orders for patients who are not in a hospice program should be reviewed by a medical professional who has not previously been directly involved with the case as a primary provider.

7. At the end of life, health care and security staff should work cooperatively to ensure that the process of dying is dignified and that policies and procedures recognize both public safety and humane prisoner treatment. Security measures (e.g., shackles) for the transportation of terminally and acutely ill patients should take into account the fragility of their physical condition. Statements of health care staff that certain standard security restraints are inappropriate to the patient's medical condition and will cause pain or further injury must be honored by security staff. Rather than developing a standardized policy on restraints, individualized assessments should be made and documented for each prisoner.

8. Advance care planning must include arrangements for timely notification of the health care proxy or other family and friends the patient wishes to be alerted when his or her condition changes or death occurs.

References

Cohn F. The ethics of end-of-life care for prison inmates. *J Law Med Ethics.* 1999;27:252-259.

Larson DG, Tobin DR. End-of-life conversations: evolving practice and theory. *JAMA.* 2000;284:1573-1578.

Parker FR, Paine CJ. Informed consent and the refusal of medical treatment in the correctional setting. *J Law Med Ethics.* 1999;27:240-251.

Chapter VII ——————————————————————

Specific Populations ——————

VII.A HEALTH SERVICES FOR WOMEN

Principle: Jail and prison health programs must provide the services and facilities necessary to meet women's health care needs, even when women are only a small proportion of the institutional population.

Public Health Rationale: Most incarcerated women are of reproductive age and have children for whom they were the primary caretaker prior to incarceration. Past abusive relationships, including childhood abuse, sexual violence, intimate partner violence, and substance abuse are common experiences in a women prisoner population. All of these features contribute to health risks such as sexually transmitted infections and other reproductive system disorders, high-risk pregnancies, chronic blood-borne infections, post traumatic stress disorder, depression, and self-harming behaviors. A good initial medical screening and complete medical examination, regular periodic screening examinations, and prevention are the hallmark of health services for women of reproductive age.

Satisfactory Compliance:
1. Initial medical screenings for women must include evaluation of the reproductive system. Special attention must also be given to any history of abusive relationships and substance misuse or abuse and treatment. Intake medical histories for incarcerated women must include questions about menses, pregnancy, contraception use, safer sex practices, reproductive system disease, and dependent children. A sensitive and dignified pelvic and breast examination must be provided as well and should include the collection of specimens for cervical cytology (Pap test), gonorrhea, chlamydia, and other vaginal infections. Instruction in self breast examination and age-appropriate mammography must also be provided.
2. Periodic reproductive system examinations, including pelvic and breast examinations, Pap tests, and mammography must be provided according to contemporary community guidelines. There must also be a system for tracking periodic examinations.

3. Gynecologic services for incarcerated women must ensure appropriate and prompt follow-up of pathology with onsite or readily available access to colposcopy and ultrasound.

4. Consideration must be given to the special dietary needs of women in menu preparation for female prisoner populations.

5. Prenatal care that is provided by professionals with training and experience in obstetrical care must begin as soon as pregnancy is identified and must meet all contemporary community standards, including appropriate screening tests, health education, and nutrition. Special housing and diets must be available for pregnant women when necessary to sustain a healthy pregnancy. High-risk pregnancies must be identified and referred appropriately. Treatment to prevent perinatal transmission of HIV must be provided to HIV-positive pregnant women and should be consistent with standards adopted by the American College of Obstetrics and Gynecology.

6. Jails and prisons must have standing arrangements for deliveries that include time for the mother and infant to be together after birth. The arrangement must allow a longer than usual stay in the hospital postpartum to provide the woman prisoner time with her infant. Women must never be shackled during labor and delivery.

7. Postpartum women must be placed in mother-infant facilities with nurseries whenever possible. Women's facilities must have provisions for infant visiting for those women who cannot be placed in mother-infant facilities.

8. Health care staff in jails and prisons housing women must be trained and prepared for labor and delivery in the event of emergencies.

9. Women prisoners must have access to family planning services, including abortion counseling and services on request.

10. Women prisoners must have access to contraception, including emergency contraception. Sterilization must only be provided with voluntary written informed consent after counseling by an outside agency and consistent with state laws. Sterilization should not follow immediately upon giving birth.

11. Hormone replacement therapy should be available when indicated.

12. Health care for incarcerated women should include services that address the consequences of abusive relationships. The safety of the women should be ensured and care should be provided for the physical and emotional sequela of abuse.

13. Sexual relationships between women prisoners and male prisoners or jail or prison staff must be considered nonconsensual and must not be tolerated. Prosecution and disciplinary action of staff involved in sexual relationships with women prisoners must be pursued. Policies must be established to minimize the risk of sexual advances on women prisoners. (e.g., male prisoner trustees must not be allowed in women's areas. Female corrections staff must be assigned to areas and tasks which involve unclothed women prisoners.)

14. Jails and prisons must work with community-based organizations to provide women prisoners with regular access to their children. Prior to visitation, prisoners should take classes on parenting education and modeling.

Social services must be available to every prisoner entering custody who is a guardian of children under the age of 18 to assure the child's welfare and protection. Counseling and assistance must also be provided to women (and men) whose legal custody of dependent children is challenged or withdrawn during incarceration.

Cross References

Access to Care, I.B
Initial Medical Screening and Complete Medical Examination, III.A
Periodic Health Assessment, III.G
Mental Health Services, V
Sexuality, VI.D
Wellness Promotion and Health Education, IX

References

Archie CL. Obstetric management of the addicted pregnant woman. In: *Drug Dependency in Pregnancy: Managing Withdrawal.* Maternal and Child Health Branch, California Department of Health Services; 1992.

Boudin K, Carrero I, Clark J, et al. ACE: a peer education and counseling program meets the needs of incarcerated women with HIV/AIDS issues. *J Assoc Nurses AIDS Care.* 1999;10:90-98.

Breuner CC, Farrow JA. Pregnant teens in prison. Prevalence, management, and consequences. *West J Med.* 1995;162:328-330.

Brewer MK, Baldwin D. The relationship between self-esteem, health habits, and knowledge of BSE practice in female inmates. *Public Health Nurse.* January-February 2000;17:16-24.

Center for Substance Abuse Treatment. CSAT releases guide for developing substance abuse treatment services for women in U.S. jails and prisons. *Psychiatr Serv.* 1999;50: 1373.

Cordero L, Hines S, Shibley KA, Landon MB. Perinatal outcome for women in prison. *J Perinatol.* 1992;12:205-209.

Fogel CI, Belyea M. The lives of incarcerated women: violence, substance abuse, and at risk for HIV. *J Assoc Nurses AIDS Care.* 1999;10:66-74.

Fogel CI, Harris BG. Expecting in prison: preparing for birth under conditions of stress. *JOGNN.* 1986;454-458.

Fogel CI. Hard time: the stressful nature of incarceration for women. *Issues Ment Health Nurs.* 1993;14:367-377.

Fogel CI. Pregnant inmates: risk factors and pregnancy outcomes. *JOGNN.* 1993;22:33-39.

Fogel CI. Health problems and needs of incarcerated women. *J Prison Jail Health.* 1991;10:45-57.

Henderson DJ. Drug abuse and incarcerated women. A research review. *J Subst Abuse Treat.* 1998;15:579-587.

Jordan BK, Schlenger WE, Fairbank JA, Caddell JM. Prevalence of psychiatric disorders among incarcerated women: convicted felons entering prison. *Arch Gen Psychiatry.* 1996;53:513-519.

Jose-Kampfner C. Reflections from the inside. Women's health in prisons. *Health PAC Bull.* 1992;22:15-19, 49.

Keaveny ME, Zauszniewski JA. Life events and psychological well-being in women sentenced to prison. *Issues Ment Health Nurs.* 1999;20:73-89.

Lindquist CH, Lindquist CA. Health behind bars: utilization and evaluation of medical care among jail inmates. *J Community Health.* 1999;24:285-303.

Martin, RE. A review of prison cervical cancer screening program in British Columbia. *Can. J. Pub. Health.* November-December 1998;89:382-86.

Pomeroy EC, Kiam R, Abel E. Meeting the mental health needs of incarcerated women. *Health Soc Work.* 1998;23: 71-75.

Richie BE, Johnsen C. Abuse histories among newly incarcerated women in a New York City jail. *JAMWA.* 1996;51:111-114, 117.

Safyer SM, Richmond L. Pregnancy behind bars. *Semin Perinatol.* 1995;19:314-322.

Smith BV, Dailard C. Female prisoners and AIDS: on the margins of public health and social justice. *AIDS Public Policy J.* 1994;9:78-85.

Teplin LA, Abram KM, McClelland GM. Prevalence of psychiatric disorders among incarcerated women: pretrial jail detainees. *Arch Gen Psychiatry.* 1996;53:505-512.

Wilson JS, Leasure R. Cruel and unusual punishment: the health care of women in prison. *Nurse Pract.* 1991;16:32,34,36-9.

Zaitzow BH. Women prisoners and HIV/AIDS. *J Assoc Nurses AIDS Care.* 1999;10:78-89.

Legal References

Doe v Barron, 92 F Supp 2d 694 (SD Oh 1999).

Coleman v Rahija, 114 F3d 778 (8th Cir 1997).

Women Prisoners of the Dist. of Columbia Dept. of Corrections, 877 F Supp 634, 666-669 (DDC 1994).

Boswell v County of Sherburne, 849 F2d 1117, 1122 (8th Cir 1988).

Mommouth Co. Correctional Institutional Inmates v Lanzaro, 834 F2d 326 (3rd Cir 1987).

Herrera v Valentine, 653 F2d 1220 (8th Cir 1981).

Todaro v Ward, 565 F2d 48, 51-52 (2nd Cir 1977).

VII.B   CHILDREN AND ADOLESCENTS

Principle: Juveniles who are incarcerated must be provided with health services appropriate to the special needs of this age group. Juveniles must be housed and treated separately from adults.

Public Health Rationale: Children and adolescents are still developing physically and mentally. They may have health problems that are different from those of adults and that require the care of physicians and other health professionals with training and experience in adolescent care. In addition, incarceration itself may have a more serious emotional impact on youth than adults.

Recent changes in judicial practices in many states have moved juveniles accused of serious felonies from family courts to criminal courts. As a result, large numbers of youth are tried as adults and sentenced to state prisons rather than juvenile justice programs. Nevertheless, children continue to have special status under the law and have rights to treatment, education, and rehabilitative programming above and beyond those required for adults.

Most incarcerated youth come from families and will return to their families after release. Family involvement in rehabilitative programming is essential, especially in mental health services.

With widespread dismantling of state mental health systems for children many juvenile justice agencies are admitting large numbers of mentally ill youth. Mental health programs must expand rapidly to meet the treatment needs of this growing segment of the population.

Youth in the justice system have substantial health needs. Dental, mental health, and substance abuse problems, including the abuse of tobacco, are widespread. Many of the most common medical problems (i.e., traumatic injuries, sexually transmitted diseases, and pregnancy) are directly related to impulsive, high-risk behaviors associated with immaturity.

Dental caries (soft, decayed area in a tooth) and fractured front teeth are the most common physical health problems among incarcerated youth. Moreover, adolescence is the age of greatest incidence of caries in the permanent molar teeth. Filling existing caries and application of pit and fissure sealants to intact molars are highly effective interventions to stop further deterioration and preserve the permanent teeth into adult life.

Asthma is the most common chronic medical condition among young people, but there are a wide variety of other chronic diseases and disabling conditions originating in childhood. For example, many of the chronic illnesses commonly associated with middle age first appear in adolescence. Early diagnosis, patient education, and effective management of diabetes, hypertension, hyperlipidemia, and smoking beginning in adolescence will prevent or reduce serious end-organ damage later in life.

Children have limited experience with and knowledge of health care issues. Emotionally immature and impulsive youth react very poorly to demands or ultimatums from institutional authorities. Health care staff needs to take a developmental approach to youth by answering questions truthfully, patiently explaining the reasons for necessary procedures or medications, and offering alternatives. It is not uncommon for a youth to adamantly refuse care at one moment and then request services a short while later.

In many cases, youth cannot provide legally adequate informed consent due to young age, immaturity, or diminished mental capacity. Special consideration must be given to issues of parental consent, confidentiality, informed consent, and the right to refuse treatment.

Satisfactory compliance:

1. All programs and health services required for adults (covered by other sections of these standards) must also be provided to juveniles.
2. All juveniles must be housed and programmed separately from adults.
3. All staff who work with youth in correctional and juvenile justice facilities must receive training on adolescent development and techniques for working effectively with young people. Of particular importance are crisis management techniques that deescalate potentially violent confrontations with impulsive youth. Training on working with mentally ill or developmentally handicapped youth and recognition of suicide risk is also required.
4. Medical programs for juveniles must be supervised by board certified physicians trained and experienced in child and adolescent medicine. Mental health programs for juveniles must be supervised by a trained and experienced child and adolescent psychiatrist.

5. There must be efforts to involve the youth's family in programming as much as possible and consistent with the needs of the youth.

6. The initial medical screening and complete medical examination must identify all health problems and result in a plan of care that includes placement in a facility with program services appropriate for the treatment and rehabilitation needs of the youth.

7. Initial medical history must include:
   a. An interview with the youth and a discussion with a parent or guardian in order to obtain more a more complete health history.
   b. Documentation of prior immunizations.
   c. History of childhood illnesses, especially chickenpox (with parental or guardian confirmation).
   d. History of major injuries including long bone fractures, head trauma with loss of consciousness, and significant wounds that may have long term residual effects.
   e. Sexual history including age of onset of sexual activity, sexual abuse, use of contraception, use of protection against HIV and other STDs, and higher risk sexual practices.
   f. Family health history with particular focus on major psychiatric illnesses, alcohol and other drug abuse problems, and significant personal losses such as separations, suicides, and other deaths.

8. The initial social history must include:
   a. Structure of the household in which the child lived and significant adult relationships, both within or outside the youth's family.
   b. Methods of parental discipline and supervision that may reveal past abuse or the origins of violent behavior or mental illness.
   c. School attendance and academic performance.

9. The initial review of systems must include inquiry about serious disorders that occur among young people including: chronic headache disorders, peptic ulcer disease, depression, sexually transmitted diseases, and cardiac problems manifested by murmurs, palpitations, chest pain, or dizziness.

10. The complete medical examination must include:
    a. Assessment of physical development by routine use of standard growth charts of height and weight percentiles for age.
    b. Assessment of sexual maturity according to the stages defined by Tanner.
    c. Scoliosis screening with particular attention to spinal curves resulting from unequal leg length.
    d. Pelvic examination must be offered and encouraged for every female, but a female prisoner's right to refuse the examination should not be denied. Pelvic examinations should be performed with patience and sensitivity by professionals who are experienced and skilled with adolescent female patients.

11. Initial screening tests must include:
    a. Formal test of hearing using a standard method with a pure tone device at selected frequencies and loudness.
    b. Formal test of vision using a standard method with a Snellen wall chart or better.

    c. Hemoglobin screening with electrophoresis to identify hemoglobins S, F, C, beta-thalassemia, or others that may have an impact on the youth's health or their childrens' health.

    d. STD screening, including syphilis serology, cervical cytology (Pap test), and tests for gonorrhea and chlamydia. Use of urine antigen amplification tests for gonorrhea and chlamydia will substantially increase the diagnosis and treatment of asymptomatic youth and reduce the reliance on painful urethral swabs to obtain a specimen.

    e. Pregnancy tests for all females.

12. The initial mental health evaluation must include:

    a. Evaluation of all youth by an experienced mental health professional with training in adolescent care.

    b. A formal mental status examination, diagnostic interview, and initial diagnostic testing.

    c. Additional specific diagnostic evaluation and testing based on initial findings of the mental health providers.

13. Immunizations must be brought up to date for age consistent with current recommendations for adolescents by the CDC, including Td (tetanus and diphtheria toxoids) booster, second MMR, hepatitis B series, hepatitis A in high-risk areas, and varicella when there is no parent confirmed history of chickenpox.

14. Other preventive services must be provided consistent with recommendations of professional organizations, such as the current American Medical Association (AMA) Guidelines for Adolescent Preventive Services.

15. Sick call and follow-up services must be available on a daily basis. Children must be given sufficient time during clinical encounters to encourage questions and permit answers that are age and language appropriate.

16. Close observation must be available for youth with evidence of suicidal risk, including arms length supervision when clinically warranted. Mentally ill youth, youth who are newly incarcerated, and youth recently adjudicated and transferred far from home are at greater risk for suicide and other self-injury behaviors. Because most successful suicides in this age group are lethal "gestures," health care, mental health, counseling, and security and supervision staff must be trained to recognize the warning signs of depression and suicide risk.

17. Mental health treatment, not limited to medication, should be provided to mentally ill, emotionally disturbed, and developmentally handicapped youth based upon the assessment and recommendations of a mental health professional. Substance abuse treatment services consistent with national standards for drug treatment should be provided to youth found to have drug abuse problems.

18. A psychiatrist trained and experienced in child and adolescent psychiatry is necessary to provide diagnosis and treatment services for youth. Other pediatric specialty services may be required to complete mental health assessments, such as for evaluation of pervasive developmental disorders.

19. Because use of psychotropic medications for adolescents is appropriate only for diagnosed psychiatric problems, the use of such medications must be

carefully monitored. Psychotropic medication should be ordered only for those children who have a diagnosed mental illness and who are managed by a psychiatrist. The use of psychotropic medication to control undisciplined youth is never appropriate nor is it permitted.

20. A formal health education program should be provided to all youth that focuses on prevention of common health issues facing young people such as sexuality and contraception, sexually transmitted diseases, HIV and AIDS, tobacco use, substance abuse, breast self-examination, testicular self-examination, and oral hygiene. These education programs should use formal curricula that have evaluated and found to be effective for young people by authorities such as the CDC's Division of Adolescent and School Health. Effective curricula that teaches skills through role playing to support behavior change should be used.

21. Facilities for youth should be tobacco free. Smoking cessation programs must be provided to youth with a history of smoking.

22. The diet for young people must provide adequate nutrients to support adolescent growth, muscle development, and youth program activities. The diet must be compatible with the Surgeon General's recommendations for a diet for all Americans and the recommended dietary allowances (RDAs) of the National Research Council for age, gender, and level of activity. In particular, nutritional analysis of facility menus by a registered dietitian must demonstrate compliance with recommendations for total calories, protein, total fat, saturated fat, cholesterol, calcium, and fiber. Fresh fruit and raw and cooked vegetables must be available daily. A system must be in place to provide extra portions to hungry youth during periods of rapid growth or increase in muscle mass.

23. An exercise program tailored to the needs and abilities of juveniles should be in place.

24. Policies and procedures must be developed that clearly outline how to handle problems and situations that arise related to:
    a. Parent or guardian consent for treatment;
    b. Confidentiality of medical and mental health information and records;
    c. Right to refuse treatment; and
    d. Forcing of treatment when there is imminent danger to self or others.

24. It is strongly recommended that juvenile facilities appoint an ombudsperson from the staff to function as a child advocate in matters that concern allegations of child abuse, inadequate medical care, and other complaints from youth.

25. Allegations of physical abuse and significant injuries of youth by staff must be reported to the state child abuse agency in order to initiate an independent investigation of possible institutional abuse.

26. Security and supervisory staff must be trained regarding the danger and recognition of restraint asphyxia that occurs when smaller youth are pinned to the ground by the weight of larger staff. All staff must be certified in cardiopulmonary resuscitation and required to initiate immediate basic life support when a youth is found to be lifeless.

Cross References

Initial Medical Screening and Complete Medical Examination, III.A
Periodic Health Assessment, III.G
Chronic Care Management, IV
Mental Health Services, V
Dental Health Care Services, VI.E
Food Services and Nutrition, VI.I
Wellness Promotion and Health Education, IX

References

American Medical Association. *Guidelines for Adolescent Preventive Services.* Chicago, Ill: American Medical Association; 1992.

Breuner CC, Farrow JA. Pregnant teens in prison. Prevalence, management, and consequences. *West J Med.* 1995;162:328-230.

Cohen MD. Special problems of health services for juvenile justice programs. In: *Clinical Practice in Correctional Medicine*, Puisis M, ed. St. Louis, Mo: Mosby Publishers; 1998.

Costello JC, Jameson EJ. Legal and ethical duties of health care professionals to incarcerated children. *Journal of Legal Medicine.* 1987;8:191-263.

Farrow JA, Schroeder E. Sexuality education groups in juvenile detention. *Adolescence.* 1984;19:817-826.

Feinstein RA, Lampkin A, Lorish CD, Klerman LV, Maisiak R, Oh MK. Medical status of adolescents at time of admission to a juvenile detention center. *J Adolesc Health.* 1998;22:190-196.

Glick B, Sturgeon W. *No Time to Play: Youthful Offenders in Adult Correctional Systems.* Washington, DC: American Correctional Association; 1998.

Jameson EJ. Incarcerated adolescents. The need for the development of professional ethical standards for institutional health care providers. *J Adolesc Health Care.* 1989;10:490-499.

Litt IF, Cohen MI. Prisons, adolescents, and the right to quality medical care: the time is now. *Am J Public Health.* 1974;64:894-897.

United States Department of Justice. *Standards for the Administration of Juvenile Justice: Report of the National Advisory Committee for Juvenile Justice and Delinquency Prevention.* Washington, DC: US Government Printing Office; 1980.

Legal References

Alexander S. v Boyd, 876 F Supp 773 (DSC 1995).

Gary H. v Hegstrom, 831 F2d 1430 (9th Cir 1987).

H.C. v. Jarrard, 786 F.2d 1080 (11th Cir 1986).

Johnson v Bell, 487 F Supp 977 (ED Mich 1980).

US ex Rel. Dancy v Arnold, 572 F2d 107 (3rd Cir 1978).

Morgan v Sproat, 432 F Supp 1130 (SD Miss 1977).

Pena v New York Sate Division for Youth, 419 F Supp 203 (SD NY 1976).

Inmates of Boys Training School v Affleck, 346 F Supp 1354 (DRI 1972).

Nelson v Heyne, 355 F Supp 451 (ND Ind 1972) *aff'd.* 419 F2d (7th Cir 1974), *cert. denied*, 417 US 976 (1974).

VII.C FRAIL-ELDERLY OR DISABLED PERSONS

Principle: Frail-elderly and disabled persons constitute a growing proportion of people in jails and prisons. Provision of adequate health care services for such groups requires special programs and resources. Clinical services and accessible and barrier-free housing must be provided and be consistent with national community standards of care and mindful of the particular legal and ethical considerations present in correctional facilities.

Public Health Rationale: The provision of adequate health and mental health services to these populations requires: 1) assessment of the health characteristics and needs of these groups within specific institutions or facilities; 2) establishment of sheltered housing and long-term care programs; and 3) when indicated, gerontologic, geriatric, rehabilitation medicine, and pain management consultation. The early identification of their needs and appropriate planning can minimize the suffering of the patients.

Satisfactory Compliance:

1. The health care system must periodically conduct (at least once every 5 years) a systematic survey to determine the size, health characteristics, and special health care needs of frail-elderly and disabled prisoners.

2. Based on the foregoing survey and other empirical information, the health care program should ascertain the scope of the need for sheltered and rehabilitative housing units and long-term care programs.

3. Prisoners who are incapacitated and who have special needs should be provided with housing and other facilities that minimize functional barriers and maximize independence. All correctional facilities must be compliant with the Americans with Disabilities Act and state and local laws, regulations, and standards regarding accessibility. These patients must also have access to the full range of program services.

4. Sheltered living units and chronic care facilities should comply with contemporary national standards of care for equivalent community facilities, either health-related or skilled nursing facilities.

5. Health care programs must conduct a formal annual audit and evaluation of health care services provided to all frail elderly, chronically-ill, and disabled persons. This evaluation must include the need for all current medications and a comprehensive assessment of functional capacity and patients' other social, emotional, and psychological needs.

6. Health care programs must maintain documentation of its activities in meeting the foregoing standards and in seeking such geriatric and rehabilitation medicine consultation as may be necessary in the development of adequate programs and services for frail-elderly, chronically ill, or disabled prisoners.

7. Facility health services must be staffed at levels that provide for assistance with daily living at the level that is required by the needs of the prisoners. Staff, not other prisoners, must be available to assist the frail-elderly and disabled prisoners. Peer support should be encouraged, but only to supplement care provided by health care staff.

Cross References

Chronic Care Management, IV

Palliative Care, Pain, and Symptom Management, VI.J

Reference

Simon S, Wilson LB, Hermalin I, Hess R, eds. *Aging and Prevention.* New York, NY: Haworth Press; 1983.

Legal References

Ancata v Prison Health Services, Inc., 769 F2d 700 (11th Cir 1985).

Balla v Idaho State Board of Corrections, 595 F Supp 1558 (D Idaho 1984).

Goodman v Wagner, 553 F Supp 255 (ED Pa 1982).

Groseclose v Dutton, 609 F Supp 1432 (MD Tenn 1985).

Hearn v Hudson, 549 F Supp 949 (WD Va 1982).

Johnson v Harris, 479 F Supp 333 (SD NY 1979).

Kahane v Carlson, 527 F2d 492 (2d Cir 1975).

McDaniel v Rhodes, 512 F Supp 117 (SD Ohio 1981).

Mitchell v Chester County Farms Prison, 426 F Supp 271 (ED Pa 1976).

Rue v Estelle, 503 F Supp 1265 (SD Tex 1980).

Villa v Franzen, 511 F Supp 231 (ND 111, 1981).

West v Keve, 517 F2d 158 (3d Cir 1978).

VII.D SEGREGATION

Principle: Medical and psychiatric services must play an important protective role in the care of segregated prisoners.

Public Health Rationale: Prisons and jails use segregated housing for three purposes: to discipline rule breakers, to protect at-risk prisoners, and to enforce administrative guidelines. Prisoners in segregation are usually confined to their cells for 22 to 23 hours per day. There are few or no congregate activities and there is little or no access to work, education, or culture. Only limited non-contact visits are allowed. While every detention facility has cells assigned for short-term segregation, since the 1970s prison systems in the United States have built free-standing long-term segregation facilities called control units or supermax units. These units provide prisoners with almost no human contact and result in increased physical and psychological morbidity.

Long-term segregated prisoners suffer from social isolation and reduced environmental stimulation. Such close confinement raises medical, psychiatric, and ethical concerns over the debilitating effects of long-term segregation and over the role of the care providers in anything but a protective function.

Satisfactory Compliance:

1. Health care staff must screen prisoners prior to their placement in segregation. Prisoners whose mental health or medical needs will be significantly compromised must be kept out of segregation.

2. Except for brief periods, all prisoners with psychiatric or mental disabilities, or who are at serious risk of injury to their mental health, must be excluded from segregated housing.

3. Prisoners in need of emergency medical, dental, or psychiatric care must be treated before they are put in segregation and they must have access to urgent and emergency care when they are in segregation.

4. Prisoners with physical disabilities must be excluded from segregation unless the cells, service routines, and attendant care meet criteria for accommodation under the Americans with Disabilities Act.

5. All prisoners confined in segregated housing must be visited by health care providers capable of assessment and triage at least once daily. A physician must make weekly rounds in all segregated areas. Health care providers must make daily log reports that include medical complaints, findings and assessment, adequacy of oral intake, and a visual assessment of the prisoner's general health and welfare. Every prisoner must receive a confidential medical and separate psychiatric assessment to determine suitability for continued segregation one month after confinement and then at least every 3 months thereafter, or more frequently if indicated by prisoner request, custodial identification, or health care/mental health provider referral.

6. Every segregated prisoner who, in the opinion of health care staff, requires examination must be brought to a clinical treatment area to receive care.

7. Those in segregation must be able to submit confidential requests for service at least 3 times a day. Custodial staff must have a clear, written procedure regarding the mechanism for receiving urgent requests for service and contacting the appropriate health care staff.

8. All medical care must be carried out under confidential and medically appropriate conditions outside of the cell in a fully and appropriately equipped setting. Access to specialty consultation should in no way be interfered with by segregated confinement. It is important that custody staff in all segregated housing units be specially trained to recognize a medical or psychiatric crisis. Custodial staff should also be evaluated periodically for stress disorders.

9. Special mention must be made concerning segregation units in women's facilities. Custody staff should observe women in all daily activities and deliver and answer requests for their most personal needs. Health care and mental health care staff must play an enhanced protective role regarding sexual abuse of women in segregation through direct questioning, examination, and observation. Health administration should request changes in policy to meet the internationally agreed upon exclusion of male custody staff from women's segregation facilities.

10. Segregated housing must conform to human rights standards concerning length of segregation, diet, access to sun, and large muscle exercise.

Cross References

Access to Care, I.B
Human Rights, I.D
Mental Health Services, V
Health Services for Women, VII.A

References

Benjamin TB, Lux K. Solitary confinement as psychological punishment. *Cal Wes Law R.* 1997;13:265-295.

Grassian S. Psychopathological effects of solitary confinement. *Am J Psychiatry.* November 1983;140:11,1450-1454.

Grassian S, Friedman N. Effects of sensory deprivation in psychiatric seclusion and solitary confinement. *Int J Law Psychiatry.* 1986;8:49-65.

Human Rights Watch. *Cold Storage: Super-Maximum Security Confinement in Indiana.* New York, NY: Human Rights Watch; 1997.

United Nations General Assembly. *Principle 3 of Principles of Medical Ethics Relevant to the Role of Health Personnel, Particularly Physicians, in the Protection of Prisoners and Detainees Against Torture and Other Cruel, Inhuman or Degrading Treatment or Punishment.* New York, NY: United Nations; 1982.

International Covenant on Civil and Political Rights, Article 10(1), G. A. res 2200A, 21 U.N. GAOR Supp. (#16) at 52; UN DocA/6316 (1966), 999 U.N.T.S. 171. And UN Human Rights Committee, General Comment 30, Article 7, ICCPR.

United Nations. *Standard Minimum Rules for Treatment of Prisoners.* New York, NY: United Nations; 1955.

The Hague. *Making Standards Work: An International Handbook on Good Prison Practice.* The Hague: Penal Reform International. 1995.

Legal References

Perri v Coughlin, 1999 US Dist LEXIS 20320 (ND NY 1999).

Ruiz v Johnson, 37 F Supp 2d 855, 907-915 (SD Texas 1999).

Buckley v Rogerson, 113 F3d 1125 (8th Cir 1998).

Simmons v Look, 154 F3d 805, 808 (8th Cir 1998).

Madrid v Gomez, 889 F Supp 1116, 1261 (ND Ca 1995).

Walker v Shansky, 28 F3d 666, 6733-674 (7th Cir 1994).

Davenport v DeRortis, 844 F2d 1310, 1316 (7th Cir), *cert. denied,* 488 US 908, 109 S Ct 260 (1988).

Meriwether v Faulkner, 821 F2d 408, 418, *cert. denied,* 484 US 935, 108 S Ct 311 (1987).

US v Michigan, 680 F Supp 928 (WD Mich 1987).

Balla v Idaho State Board of Corrections, 595 F Supp 1558, 1577 (D Idaho 1984).

Burks v Teasdale, 492 F Supp 650 (WD Mo1980).

Negron v Preiser, 382 F Supp 535 (SD NY 1975).

VII.E   TRANSGENDERED PERSONS

Principle: Transgendered individuals have special health and housing needs and must be offered additional health care services.

Public Health Rationale: Transgendered persons using hormonal reassignment of gender require maintenance of their medications upon arrival in prison or jail as well as regular monitoring. Many transgendered individuals have distinctive mental health needs arising from gender dysphoria, stigma, and marginality. In addition, transgenders may be subjected to violence, including rape, by other prisoners. For those transgenders already using hormonal sex reassignment, interruption of hormones can produce a rapid change in appearance, psychological, and emotional mental health. Adequate health care requires assessment and maintenance of a hormonal treatment plan, availability of mental health services, and establishment of appropriate and safe housing.

Satisfactory Compliance:

1. Health care services for transgenders must be provided by health care providers who have been trained in assessment and in monitoring hormonal supplements. An outside specialist must be available to jail- or prison-based health care staff. Hormone maintenance can be a key element in the mental health of a person who has been receiving it as part of sex reassignment.

2. Correctional officers, health care, and mental health staff at the jail or prison must be trained to understand the psychosocial and biological issues of the transgender community. Where possible support groups should be available to transgenders.

3. Prisoners must receive housing assignments that acknowledge their social and personal identity. This may be a special unit that is offered with the consent of the prisoner. Prisoners in such a unit should be able to participate in the full range of institutional programs.

4. A strong policy protecting transgenders from sexual assault, physical and verbal abuse, and discrimination should be issued. Strip searching of male-to-female (MTF) transgender prisoners by male correction officers is a violation of privacy.

5. HIV/AIDS education must be tailored to the particular needs of the transgender population.

References

San Francisco Department of Public Health. Tom Waddell Health Center Protocols for Hormonal Reassignment of Gender.

Bockting MD, Coleman E. *Gender Dysphoria: Interdisciplinary Approaches in Clinical Management.* Binghamptom, NY: Haworth Press; 1992.

Israel GE, Tarver D. *Transgender Care.* Atlanta, Ga: Temple University Press; 1997.

Kirk S. *Physician's Guide to Transgender Medicine.* Blawnox, Pa: Together Lifeworks;1996.

Kirk S. Rathblatt M. *Medical, Legal and Workplace Issues for the Transsexual.* Blawnox, Pa: Together Lifeworks;1996.

Legal References

Brown v Zavares, 63 F3d 967 (10th Cir 1995).

Taylor v Michigan Dept. of Corrections, 69 F3d 76 (6th Cir 1995).

Farmer v Haas, 990 F2d 319, 321 (7th Cir 1993).

Phillips v Michigan Dep't of Corrections, 731 F Supp 792, 794 (WD Mich 1990), *aff'd* 932 F2d 969 (6th Cir 1991).

Brown v Zavares, 63 F3d 967 (10th Cir 1995).

Meriwether v Faulkner, 821 F2d 408, 418, *cert. denied,* 484 US 935 (1987).

Supre v Ricketts, 792 F2d 958 (10th Cir 1986).

Lamb v Maschner, 633 F Supp 351 (D Kan 1986).

Chapter VIII ───────────────────

Restraints Administered by Health Care Providers ──

Principle: Physical restraints include both mechanical devices and drugs to control behavior or to restrict the patient's freedom of movement. The patient has the right to be free from restraints of any form that are not medically necessary or are used as a means of coercion, discipline, convenience, or retaliation by the medical or mental health care staff. Restraints must only be used by health care staff in emergency situations if needed to prevent prisoners from harming themselves or others, and even then they should be used only for the shortest time possible and with the least restriction possible. The need to use medical restraints is an indication that acute psychiatric hospitalization is required.

Public Health Rationale: Hundred of deaths are caused by the use of physical restraints; however, the risk of death is a function of the length of time the restraints are applied. Except in emergency situations, patient autonomy is destroyed by the use of restraints. The use of restraints by health or mental health staff should be instituted only when all other attempts to calm the prisoner have failed and when, in the judgment of a psychiatrist or physician, the threat of serious injury to self and others is so severe as to warrant such a response. Restraints should only be used in the infirmary or hospital setting for medical reasons. Restraints cannot be used because a patient refuses treatment.

Satisfactory Compliance: Written guidelines should be developed for the use of restraints that incorporate the following requirements:

1. The use of restraints must be in accordance with the order of a physician or other *licensed independent provider* and may never be written as a standing or as needed (prn) order.
2. There is no clinical situation that calls for the routine use of restraints. Suicidal prisoners should not be restrained except in emergency situations and when no less restrictive alternative is available.
3. Restraints must be applied as humanely as possible and the level of restraint should be reduced as quickly as possible to the level of least restriction necessary to protect the prisoner and others as determined by a psychiatrist.

4. The condition of the restrained patient must be continually assessed, monitored, and reevaluated. There must be documentation by health care or mental health care staff of the status of the patient at least every 15 minutes. Vital signs must be taken and recorded at least hourly.

5. A physician must see the patient and evaluate the need for restraint within 1 hour after the initiation of this intervention.

6. Orders must be limited to a period of 4 hours for adults.

7. Orders for adolescents between 9 and 17 years of age must be limited to 2 hours.

8. Once the original order expires, a physician must see and assess the patient before a new order is issued. Only one renewal is permissible. If restraint continues to be necessary, the patient must be transported to an acute hospital setting.

9. Prisoners in restraints should be allowed bathroom privileges as soon as it is practical.

10. The type of medical or therapeutic restraints accepted for similar restraint in the community should be used in the jail and prison settings. Soft restraints (e.g., canvass and fleece-lined leather) should be used. The use of metal or hard plastic cuffs would be inappropriate and should not be used for medical restraints. Prisoners being restrained by medical or mental health care staff should be restrained in positions that are acceptable in the community. The least restrictive means of restraint should be used.

11. All situations resulting in the use of physical restraints should be reviewed through the quality improvement process. Inappropriate use of restraints should be identified and sanctioned.

Cross References

Ethical and Legal Issues, I.C
Mental Health Services, V

References

Annas GJ. The last resort—the use of physical restraints in medical emergencies. *N Engl J Med.* 1998;341:1408-1412.

Legal References

Buckley v Rogerson, 133 F3d 1125 (8th Cir 1998).
Burks v Teasdale, 492 F Supp 650, 679 (WD Mo 1980).
Eckerhart v Hensley, 475 F Supp 908 (WD Mo1979).
Negron v Preiser, 382 F Supp 535, 543 (SDNY 1974).

Chapter IX ─────────────────

Wellness Promotion and Health Education ─────

IX.A INJURIES

A. Violence

Principle: It is the correctional administration's responsibility to prevent and reduce the risk and occurrence of fatal and non-fatal intentional injuries among prisoners, staff, and the community at large.

Public Health Rationale: Violence or intentional injury is a leading cause of death and disability among adolescents and young adults in the United States. Populations at risk for incarceration (e.g., poor, minorities, urban) have increased risk for death and disability from homicide and assault. In large urban centers, most homicide victims and perpetrators had prior involvement in the criminal justice system. Non-fatal violence, including rape, and aggressive physical response to conflict from prisoners and correctional staff dominate the prison experience. Restraints, including mechanical and chemical (i.e., lacrimatory agents and pepper spray) are common responses to prison violence, but can be misused or contribute to injury. The risk of fatal violence decreases while a person is incarcerated but rises rapidly upon release. Identifying risk factors for violence-related injuries and responding with appropriate prevention strategies will reduce the risk of violence to the prisoner population and, ultimately, the community upon their release.

Satisfactory Compliance:

1. Intake screening questions must include inquiries about prior violence-related injuries, including gunshot wounds, stab wounds, and assaults by an intimate partner.
2. Health care and security staff must collaborate on the surveillance of violent injuries, including injuries by staff. Security staff must investigate each incident and provide protection for the involved prisoners. Health care providers must examine every prisoner who is subjected to force or violence. The results of the examination must be kept in the health record. There should be an appeal mechanism when there is disagreement among staff about excessive force or staff involvement in violent injuries.

3. Inappropriate use of mechanical and chemical restraints must be documented as excessive force. Health care staff must document and report abuses with restraints.

4. Health care surveillance should assist in the development of corrective action plans based on patterns of increased violent or suspected violent injury and any events of excessive use of force by staff.

5. Facilities should maintain a separate file of all injuries that are maintained for statistical purposes (e.g., trend and pattern analysis). This file should consist of anonymous aggregate data separate from health records.

6. Care for an intentional injury must be supportive and nonjudgmental. Mental health counseling must be available to assault victims.

7. Health education and prevention counseling must incorporate information about reducing the risk of violence, such as the health risks associated with firearms or abusive relationships. Efforts should be intensified for persons with identified risk factors such as prior victimization, repeated incarcerations, gang membership, or history of witnessing violent events.

8. Rape and other sexual assault victims must have access to specialized rape examinations and counseling services. Collaboration with community-based providers is encouraged.

9. Staff training must include policies about the management of injuries (including but not limited to the requirement to treat injured prisoners with dignity and respect) and the handling of bodily fluid exposures. There must also be training about the use of mechanical and chemical restraints, including documentation of their use and misuse. Lacrimatory agents and pepper spray must never be used in confined spaces.

B.   Unintentional Injuries

Principle: It is the responsibility of the correctional administration to prevent and reduce the risk of fatal and non-fatal unintentional injuries among prisoners and to minimize prolonged disability when injuries occur.

Public Health Rationale: Injury is a common but preventable health problem in jails and prisons and can result in permanent disability or death. Prevalent unintentional injuries among incarcerated populations occur during recreation or work. These include injury due to cold, excessive heat, and unsafe equipment. Such injuries can be reduced or prevented by environmental controls and proper training and equipment.

Satisfactory Compliance:
1. There must be surveillance of unintentional injuries. Corrective action plans must be developed for patterns of increased injury.

2. Care for injuries must be directed toward minimizing prolonged or permanent disability.

3. Safe environments, proper equipment, and training must be provided to minimize the risk of unintentional injuries.

IX.B OCCUPATIONAL HEALTH

Principle: It is the responsibility of correctional administrators and industry managers to prevent workplace injuries and illness.

Public Health Rationale: Workplace safety and health in the public and private sectors is within the jurisdiction of federal and state regulatory agencies. These agencies promulgate and are responsible for enforcing extensive and comprehensive standards concerning potentially dangerous working conditions. The employment of prisoners in correctional institutions involves hazards identical or similar to those faced by non-institutionalized workers who perform the same jobs. It follows, therefore, that the same health and safety standards that are applicable to non-incarcerated workers must be applied to prisoner labor, whether the work is done within the jails and prisons, or in the community.

Satisfactory Compliance:

1. Manufacturing, service, construction, and agricultural activities must comply with all federal and state standards for hazard abatement.
2. There must be regular inspections of prisoner work sites by a trained, qualified professional to ensure that health and safety standards are met. These inspectors must have the authority to mandate modifications to abate hazards.
3. Prisoners must receive adequate and appropriate training to carry out their assigned tasks and the training must be documented. They must be provided with appropriate equipment and work must be supervised by persons knowledgeable about workplace safety.
4. The safe handling of toxic chemicals must be ensured by training and ready access of the Material Safety Data Sheets.
5. Health care staff must collaborate with prison industry staff to carry out occupational injury surveillance. Corrective action plans must be developed for patterns of injuries.
6. Health care staff must screen prisoners to determine any limitations to work assignments and performance.

IX.C HEALTH EDUCATION AND HEALTH PROMOTION

Principle: Informed, educated patients are best equipped to participate in the treatment of their illnesses, maintenance of health, and recognition and prevention of potential problems. Health information provides every individual with a measure of control and self-determination, feelings that are particularly important for the incarcerated. Well-planned preventive health and health promotion programs contribute to the health and well-being of the entire prison population and must be available in every jail and prison.

Public Health Rationale: Health education and promotion are key strategies to improve the health and well-being of individuals and populations. The focus is prevention—the cornerstone of public health. Prison populations are comprised of groups that suffer health disparities in the community. Poverty and discrimination contribute to the disproportionate ill health of these groups. Effective health education and promotion can help close the gap in health outcome in these populations by preventing or improving behaviors, environmental impacts, and other unhealthy determinants that are prevalent in the communities from which many prisoners come.

Regular and culturally competent communication between health care provider and patient must be the generally accepted and practiced policy of the health care program. Such communication is the primary element of adequate health education. Jail and prison health care staffs often have the opportunity to be the first to instruct and to discuss health needs with patients, many of whose lives have not provided them with environments in which such information or attention is available. Peer education has also been found to be a very effective means of teaching people about important health topics and should be supported and used in jail and prison settings. In addition, while prisoners spend longer time in custody, new information becomes available that may not have been available to them before.

Satisfactory Compliance:

1. There must be a health education program at every jail and prison facility, which through structured and sustained efforts has as its goal improving prisoner health by developing sound health practices, attitudes, habits, and behaviors. For the most effective communication of health information, a wide variety of educational approaches should be utilized. These may include peer education, lecture-discussion formats, "rap" sessions, role-playing, storytelling, audiovisual presentations, and current health literature. Health information must include the following topics:
   a. Mental health (including personality development and stress management);
   b. Drug use and abuse (alcohol included);
   c. Tobacco;
   d. Injury and violence prevention;
   e. Family living and human sexuality (including information on contraception, sexually transmitted diseases, rape, and relationship abuse, including child and partner abuse);
   f. Nutrition, diet, and weight control;
   g. Disease prevention and control, including information on health maintenance and symptoms of common diseases, information and support groups for prisoners with chronic diseases (i.e., diabetes, asthma, HIV, heart disease, hypertension), self-examinations for disease detection (i.e., breast exam and testicular self-exam), and infectious diseases (especially venereal disease, hepatitis, tuberculosis, upper respiratory infection, skin infestation), and information about tattooing and its complications;
   h. Special concerns of women prisoners (e.g., menstruation, pregnancy, pre- and postnatal care, menopause);
   i. Personal hygiene;
   j. Safety and first aid (i.e., information on cardiopulmonary resuscitation);
   k. Physical fitness and cardiovascular/pulmonary health;
   l. Dental health; and
   m. Discharge planning.
2. Patients must always know their medical diagnoses and the names of the medications they take. Patients who want a list of medications with instruc-

tions must be given such information along with counseling regarding the possible difficulties that having such written information may pose to its confidentiality. The medications must be reviewed at every medical interaction. Ultimately, the patient will probably travel without the medical record and must have no confusion about medications, doses, and past medical history.

3. Clear, written health information that is in appropriate and culturally competent language for the population and geared to the general educational level of the prisoner population, as well as verbal information, must be available in the prison library and the clinic for prisoners who are interested in knowing more about their health conditions. This information must include listings of potential resources for follow-up care after discharge when feasible. Health care staff must have access to current information for staff and prisoners regarding all health care topics.

IX.D HEALTH MAINTENANCE AND EXERCISE

Principle: Health care programs in jails and prisons must provide for the diagnosis and treatment of illness, but also must include organized programs of health maintenance and disease prevention.

Public Health Rationale: The adequacy of any organized health care program, whether in a correctional institution or elsewhere, resides not only in the diagnosis and treatment of disease but also in the application of knowledge that maintains health and prevents disease. Maintenance of health and prevention of disease can be accomplished through programs of health education and by health screening performed according to established protocols. Proper nutrition, availability of aerobic exercise, environmental safety, and programs to aid smoking cessation also are crucial elements of an adequate health maintenance component of health services in correctional institutions.

Satisfactory Compliance:

1. Health services programs must have a set of written policies and procedures that define the components of the institution's health maintenance activities.

2. Health maintenance activities must include a formal health education program that provides information concerning nutrition and exercise and the health effects of tobacco, alcohol, and drug abuse.

3. In any institution in which prisoners are confined for 1 or more months, the health service must provide medical assistance and counseling to prisoners wishing to discontinue use of tobacco. Such assistance should be documented in a written protocol.

4. Institutions must provide nonsmoking prisoners with an environment that eliminates the detrimental health effects of passive tobacco smoke.

5. All institutions must provide access to an area outside the living area suitable for 1 hour of large muscle aerobic exercise 7 days per week. Except under extreme climatic conditions, available exercise areas must include outside facilities that permit regular exposure to sunlight.

Cross References

Environmental Health, X

References

Injuries

Morrison EF. Victimization in prison: implications for the mentally ill inmate and for health professionals. *Arch Psychiatr Nurs.* 1991;5:17-24.

May JP, Lambert WL. Preventive health issues for individuals in jails and prisons. In: *Clinical Practice in Correctional Medicine.* Puisis M, ed. St. Louis, Mo: Mosby Publishers; 1998:259-274.

Health Education and Health Promotion

Centers for Disease Control and Prevention. HIV/AIDS education and prevention programs for adults in prisons and jails and juveniles in confinement facilities—United States, 1994. *JAMA.* 1996;275:1306-1308.

Centers for Disease Control and Prevention. HIV/AIDS education and prevention programs for adults in prisons and jails and juveniles in confinement facilities—United States, 1994. *MMWR Morb Mortal Wkly Rep.* 1996;45:268-71.

Boudin K, Carrero I, Clark J, et al. ACE: a peer education and counseling program meets the needs of incarcerated women with HIV/AIDS issues. *J Assoc Nurses AIDS Care.* 1999;10:90-98.

Dolan KA, Wodak AD, Hall WD. A bleach program for inmates in NSW: an HIV prevention strategy. *N Z J Pub Health.* December 1998;22:838-840.

King L, Coleman T, Whitman S. The smoking habits of prisoners: the synergetic price of incarceration. Paper presented at: Sixth National Conference on Medical Care and Health Services in Correctional Institutions; October 9, 1982; Chicago, Ill.

Taylor RB, ed. *Health Promotion: Principles and Clinical Applications.* Norwalk, Conn: Appleton Century-Crofts; 1982.

United States Public Health Service. A clinical practice guideline for treating tobacco use and dependence. *JAMA.* June 2000;283:3244-3254.

Health Maintenance and Exercise

Thomas G, Lee PR, Franks P, Paffenbarger RS. *Exercise and Health: The Evidence and the Implications.* Cambridge, Mass: Oelgeschlager, Gunn & Hain Publishers, Inc.; 1981.

Legal References

Hemmings v Gorczyk, 134 F3d 104 (2nd Cir 1998).

Watson v Caton, 984 F2d 537 (8th Cir 1993).

Wooten v US, 825 F2d 1039 (6th Cir 1987).

Chapter X ──────────────────────────

Environmental Health ──────

Principle: Most environmental health standards are facility related. For example, as prisoners move through the correctional system, they are housed in facilities ranging from very restrictive maximum security cells to residential dwellings where they have mobility. In each case, the environmental health needs of prisoners are comparable to those of other populations in the general community. However, the provision of those needs will be affected by the housing conditions and the level of security and the environmental health standards will vary accordingly. The standards in this book are directed toward those facilities in which mobility of prisoners is significantly restricted and the prisoner is dependent upon the facility and its staff for the provision of his or her health and safety needs.

The design, construction, operation, and maintenance of correctional facilities must comply with applicable codes, standards, rules, and regulations, particularly in the areas of building construction, accessibility, fire, safety, plumbing, water supply, wastewater disposal, air pollution control, hazardous materials and waste management, and food service. Technical information and consultations are generally available through various federal, state, and local units of government and such consultation and cooperation as may be available should be used.[1]

X.A GROUNDS AND STRUCTURES

A. Construction, Planning, and Design of Facilities

Principle: Construction and remodeling projects must comply with applicable building codes, regulations, and the satisfactory compliance issues specified in this chapter.

Public Health Rationale: The preparation and review of construction plans and specifications are next in importance to site selection in determining a healthful

───────────

1 Because environmental health concerns in correctional facilities are similar in many respects to those of other institutions, many existing standards of practice are applicable to this setting. To draft an entirely new set of standards and explanations for this special group of institutions would be repetitive and is deemed unwarranted. Therefore, reference will be freely made to applicable nationally recognized standards, codes, and regulations.

institutional environment. Careful work when planning the facility assures compliance with these and related standards and will prevent unfavorable situations from developing and costly alterations after the building has been erected and roads and utilities have been installed.

Satisfactory Compliance:

1. Plans and specifications for new construction or remodeling projects must be prepared by a registered architect or engineer. Plans must comply with applicable building codes, laws, rules, and regulations and must be approved by the appropriate federal, state, and/or local agencies prior to advertising for bids and prior to construction. Plans and specifications must consider the environmental impact of proposed structures, locations, facilities, and services. Consideration must be given to other factors including: geographic and climatic conditions, accessibility, and use; availability of municipal services, including details concerning water supply and sewage and wastewater collection, treatment, and disposal; solid waste collection, storage, and disposal; power source; heating and ventilation; air pollution control; drainage and flood control; accessibility for prisoners and staff with disabilities; food service; laundry; housing and space requirements; construction materials and maintenance; selection of equipment (i.e., food service equipment); and other specifications covered by this section. Governmental agencies (local, state, and federal) that may have a role in the review of the project or in providing a community service must be involved early in the planning. The local or state public health agency must also be involved in planning the facility.

2. Qualified environmental health staff must review and evaluate plans for the construction of proposed correctional institutions as well as additions to and rehabilitation of old facilities. Necessary approvals and consultations must be obtained from regulatory agencies that have particular expertise or jurisdiction.

B. Construction Materials and Maintenance

Principle: Construction materials must be sound and suitable for the intended use.

Public Health Rationale: The use of fire-resistant construction materials and finishes will retard the spread of fire. Construction materials and finishes must minimize the formation of toxic and asphyxiating gases in case of fire. Asbestos in surface finishes and materials may deteriorate with age and release hazardous particles and therefore must not be used. The provision of suitable surfaces that are readily cleanable and moisture resistant will prevent or reduce algal, microbial, and fungal growths and will enhance sanitary maintenance. Consideration of noise and vibration control in building design and material selection will minimize problems associated with noise-related stress and assure greater compliance with noise level standards. Community standards must be met regardless of state exemptions for state constructed buildings.

Satisfactory Compliance:

1. Construction materials must comply with the standards established in state or nationally recognized building, fire prevention, plumbing, electrical,

mechanical, and sanitary codes and be maintained in compliance with such codes and used for the intended purpose. Surfaces are painted or finished in a manner appropriate to assure compliance with fire safety and cleanability requirements.

2. For existing facilities, a survey must be made to identify the presence of asbestos surfaces and materials, and a plan must be implemented to remove or protect hazardous surfaces and materials in accordance with federal standards—National Institute for Occupational Safety and Health (NIOSH), Occupational Safety and Health Administration (OSHA), and the Environmental Protection Agency (EPA).

3. All structural and mechanical equipment must be maintained in satisfactory condition by a preventive maintenance program that includes scheduled inspection of the building and inspection and maintenance of all mechanical equipment. Dates of inspections and equipment services and corrective actions must be recorded and maintained for at least 2 years.

C. Drainage and Protection from Flooding and Other Natural Disasters

Principle: Structures and facilities must not be located in areas subject to flooding or in areas that have inadequate drainage.

Public Health Rationale: Construction of facilities above flood plain levels and on well-drained land will reduce the risk of flood damage and help control the spread of vector-borne diseases. Proper drainage will also reduce facility and equipment failures and operational problems associated with periodic flooding. Such failures may have negative consequences for the health and safety of prisoners and personnel.

Satisfactory Compliance: Structures and facilities must not be located in areas designated as flood plains by the US Army Corps of Engineers or other official agencies. Areas that collect water must be drained, and culverts and ditches must be adequate to prevent ponding or flooding.

D. Highways, Access Roads, Service Entrances, and Traffic Safety

Principle: Highways and internal roads should provide safe and convenient ingress to and egress from the institution. Roads within the complex must be properly designed, illuminated, marked, and maintained to ensure safe use.

Public Health Rationale: Properly designed, illuminated, marked, and maintained roads will reduce vehicular injuries and help save lives.

Satisfactory Compliance:

1. Road intersections, speed limits, and hazardous locations should be marked and illuminated. Road widths, shoulders, grades, and lines of sight should be adequate for the expected vehicular and pedestrian traffic. Ready access should be available for emergency vehicles and staff, should an incident occur. Separate lanes should be provided to permit safe exit from or entrance to highways. Intersections and other natural or man-made hazards should be properly marked and illuminated with advance warning markers or signs. Road design, construction, and markings should comply with applicable

state or federal standards. Traffic regulations within the correctional complex must be enforced.

2. Access roads and service entrances must be safe, convenient for emergency vehicle use, and adequate for their intended purpose. They must be of such design, width, and grade as to minimize accidents, facilitate ingress and egress, and permit ready use and turnaround by private and commercial vehicles (including street cleaners, snow plows, fire trucks, and service vehicles) without impeding traffic. Vehicles used to transport prisoners must have restraint systems. Vehicles that transport wheelchair-bound prisoners must be appropriately equipped to provide safe transport for such prisoners.

3. Loading docks and other areas with heavy vehicular traffic must not be located in proximity to fresh air inlets for the HVAC systems or to operable windows of prisoner cells, day rooms, or other habitable areas.

E.   Location and Accessibility of Service Areas

Principle: Attention to safety principles must be applied in the location, design, and maintenance of facilities and services. This should include provision of safe ingress to and egress from the facility.

Public Health Rationale: Facility location, design, and maintenance may affect prisoner health and safety through impact on disease transmission, fires, accidents, and effects of natural disasters. The design, location, and maintenance of interior roads and service entrances are critical in the event of internal disasters.

Satisfactory Compliance: All structures and facilities (such as prisoner- and staff-occupied buildings, power plants, fire stations, water plants, water towers, solid waste facilities, sewage treatment facilities, and pumping stations) must be located on stable ground and should meet applicable community codes and standards for design, maintenance, and operation.

Legal References

Tillery v Owens, 907 F2d 418, 422 (3rd Cir 1990).
Hoptowit v Spellman, 753 F2d 779, 784 (9th Cir 1985).
Jones v City & Co. of SF, 976 F Supp 896, 909 (ND Ca 1997).
Carty v Farrelly, 957 F Supp 727 (DVI 1997).
Hendrix v Faulkner, 525 F Supp 435 (ND Ind 1981).
Grubbs v Bradley, 552 F Supp 1052 (MD Tenn 1980).
Feliciano v Barcelo, 497 F Supp 14, 20 (DPR 1979).

X.B   SERVICES AND UTILITIES

A.   Air Quality

Principle: Unhealthful airborne chemicals and respirable and nonrespirable particulates must be controlled at safe levels, as defined by national and local community environmental health standards. In addition, indoor air must be free of objectionable odors.

Emissions from facility operations must not exceed minimum standards of the EPA and OSHA, or applicable state standards.

Public Health Rationale: Ventilation and clean air are necessary for a healthy environment. Indoor and outdoor air pollutants have been shown to cause or aggravate respiratory disease and to cause nausea, headaches, eye irritation, and allergies.

Satisfactory Compliance:

1. Mechanical ventilation systems must provide a minimum air supply of 20 cubic feet per minute (cfm) per person of outside air, or recirculated filtered air, to the cellblocks per current American Society of Heating, Refrigerating, and Air-Conditioning Engineers (ASHRAE) standards.[2] Approximately one third of the recirculated air should be fresh outside air. Fresh air inlets should be installed isolated from loading areas and other possible sources of air contaminants.

2. Workplace-related exposures to airborne contaminants must meet OSHA standards. Appropriate air flow and local exhaust capacity must be provided to assure that concentrations of harmful chemical vapors and gases or respirable dusts do not exceed OSHA standards. The institution must have a policy designating smoking and nonsmoking environments.

3. All facility operations must comply with performance and emission standards as defined by state and federal agencies, including installation and operation permits, where applicable. Pollution control equipment must be used and maintained to minimize deterioration of the environment and harmful exposures to people. Staff operators must be trained in proper maintenance and operations of equipment. They are instructed to contact the appropriate federal, state, or local pollution control agency whenever equipment malfunctions may lead to air pollution. Operator training programs must be documented.

4. When air pollution prevention is based upon fuel specifications, such as low sulfur content fuel, samples of the fuel, as delivered, must be analyzed by a qualified laboratory.

Legal References

Helling v McKinney, 509 US 25, 25, 113 S Ct 2475 (1993).
Keenan v Hall, 83 F3d 1083 (9th Cir 1995).
Tillery v Owens, 907 F2d 418, 423 (3rd Cir 1990).
Cody v Hillard, 599 F Supp 1025 (SDSD 1984), aff'd by 799 F2d 447 (8th Cir 1986).
Hoptowit v Spellman, 753 F2d 779, 784 (9th Cir 1985).
Jones v City & Co. of SF, 976 F Supp 896, 912-913 (ND Ca 1997).

B.   Temperature, Humidity, and Ventilation Control

Principle: HVAC control systems must be properly designed, operated, and maintained to provide a healthful environment. A control system requires consideration of ambient air temperature, air movement, and relative humidity.

Public Health Rationale: Adequate control systems are necessary to assure in each habitable room an indoor environment with temperature and humidity levels adequate to protect the health and comfort of all occupants.

---

2 At the time of this writing, the relevant ASHRAE standard is 62-89R.

Satisfactory Compliance:

1. In hot and dry climates, exterior window shields, shutters, or awnings must be provided to exclude solar radiation.

2. In hot and humid climates when the facility does not have mechanical chilled-air systems, adequate windows and wall openings should be provided and the location must provide cross-ventilation. Where ventilation is dependent on exterior wall openings, such openings should equal at least one-eighth (12.5%) of the floor space of the sleeping, living, educational, and work areas. Gyms and swimming pools require special temperature, humidity, and ventilation controls. Mechanical ventilation systems must provide sufficient outdoor air to meet current ASHRAE standard 62-89 or its successor.

3. The building design, insulation, and exterior surface and color minimize heat absorption. For new construction, the ASHRAE energy construction standards must be met.

4. Clothes, towels, sheets, draperies, posters, and other objects should not interfere with air flow in or out of living areas.

5. The control system should maintain an indoor air temperature of at least 68°F during the coldest months. Prisoners must not be required to perform strenuous physical activity when temperature and humidity levels meet or exceed the following standard:

Temperature (°F)	Relative Humidity (%)
95	55
96	52
97	49
98	45
99	42

6. When indoor air temperatures exceed 90°F, special precautions must be taken to ensure that prisoners are provided with extra showers, access to cool water to drink, and other appropriate measures. Special attention must be taken to protect prisoners taking medications that limit their capacity to tolerate excessive heat.

See ASHRAE Fundamentals of Ventilation Handbook; The ASHRAE Energy Conservation in New Buildings Design Standard 90-75; ASHRAE Standard 62-89R, Natural and Mechanical Ventilation; and ANSI/ASHRAE Standard 55-181, Thermal Environmental Conditions for Human Occupancy.

Legal References

Dixon v Gomez, 114 F3d 640, 663-664 (7th Cir 1997).
Mitchell v Maynard, 80 F3d 1433, 1442 (10th Cir 1996).
Keenan v Hall, 83 F3d 1083 (9th Cir 1995).
Williams v Griffin, 952 F2d 820 (4th Cir 1991).
Tillery v Owens, 907 F2d 418, 423 (3rd Cir 1990).
Hassine v Jeffes, 846 F2d 169, 174 (3rd Cir 1988).
Hoptowit v Spellman, 753 F2d 779, 784 (9th Cir 1985).
Cody v Hillard, 599 F Supp 1025 (SDSD 1984), *aff'd by* 799 F2d 447 (8th Cir 1986).
Ramos v Lamm, 639 F2d 559, 568 (10th Cir 1980), *cert. denied,* 450 US 1041, (1981).

Anton v Sheriff of Dupage Co., 47 F Supp 2d 993 (ND Ill 1999).
Blackiston v Vaughn, 1998 US Dist LEXIS 15008 (ED Pa 1998).
Jones v City & Co. of SF, 976 F Supp 896, 912-913 (ND Ca 1997).
Grubbs v Bradley, 552 F Supp 1052 (MD Tenn 1982).
Hendrix v Faulkner, 525 F Supp 435, 525-526 (ND Ind 1981).
Lightfoot v Walker, 486 F Supp 504 (SD Ill 1980).
Laaman v Helgemoe, 437 F Supp 269 (DNH 1977).
Coldsby v Carnes, 365 F Supp 395, 401-402 (WD Mo 1973).

C. Electrical Power Supply

Principle: The electrical system must be designed to meet the peak-use demand loads and have sufficient standby emergency power to maintain essential services as may be required for security, health and safety, and fire protection. Equipment and devices must be safe for use.

Public Health Rationale: Properly designed and maintained power systems are necessary to maintain essential services such as heating, air conditioning, refrigeration, lighting, elevator, and security systems. Such services are necessary to maintain comfort, provide safe storage for perishable food items and medical supplies, and support a safe environment.

Satisfactory Compliance:

1. Electrical equipment (where appropriate) must be approved by Underwriters Laboratory (UL). Electrical wiring for equipment must conform to the Underwriters Electrical Code for material, installation, and workmanship. Unless double insulated, all electrical equipment must be grounded. Electrical systems must conform to current National Fire Protection Association (NFPA) National Electrical Code, or equivalent local or state electrical code.
2. Staff operators and maintenance personnel must be trained in proper maintenance and operation of systems, detection of malfunctions, and emergency procedures.
3. Emergency power generator(s) or battery packs, when required for essential services, must be constructed, installed, and maintained to activate automatically in the event of a power failure. They must have sufficient capacity to operate electrical locking devices and other essential electrical equipment including elevators, life-sustaining medical care equipment, refrigerators and freezers, emergency lighting circuits, alarms, and communication systems for a minimum of 24 hours. The facility must also have a plan for resupply.

Legal Reference

Hendrix v Faulkner, 525 F Supp 435, 525-526 (ND Ind 1981).

D. Housekeeping

Principle: Jails and prisons must be maintained in a clean, orderly condition and be in good repair.

Public Health Rationale: Soiled walls, floors, ceilings, and fixtures and the accumulation of litter, dust, and dirt provide breeding places for disease vectors such as flies, roaches, and rodents. In addition, unsanitary conditions favor the growth or survival of disease-causing microorganisms. A clean environment helps promote personal hygiene as well as good physical and emotional health. Poor housekeeping results in accidents, creates fire hazards, and spreads disease.

Satisfactory Compliance:

1. All floors, walls, ceilings, light fixtures, equipment, and interior and exterior spaces must be kept clean and in good repair. Coving must be provided at the juncture of interior walls and floors. Cleaning equipment and facilities, including service sinks, floor drains, and storage spaces must be adequate for the tasks. A custodial sink must be available on each floor for housekeeping operations. Floors, walls, ceilings, sanitary fixtures, equipment, and facilities must be designed of easily cleanable materials. A written policy must document daily housekeeping requirements.

2. Housekeeping materials, including detergents and other indicated chemical compounds, must be properly labeled and stored. Prisoners must have cleaning items available to them (at specified intervals and not less than weekly) so that prisoners may clean their cells or living areas. Non-caustic cleaning supplies must be provided. If due to security concerns or disability of the prisoner it is not possible for a prisoner to clean his or her cell or living area, the department of corrections must make arrangements to have it cleaned at least once each week, or more often in the event of unsanitary or unsafe conditions.

3. Walks and exterior areas used for recreation must be free of debris, ice, and snow. Exterior areas, particularly walkways, must be surfaced with concrete, asphalt, gravel, or similar material to facilitate maintenance and cleanliness and to minimize dust.

Legal References

Tillery v Owens, 907 F2d 418, 423 (3rd Cir 1990).
Martin v Sargent, 780 F2d 1334, 1338 (8th Cir 1985).
Hoptowit v Spellman, 752 F2d 779, 784 (9th Cir 1985).
Ramos v Lamm, 639 F2d 559, 570 (10th Cir 1980).
Roop v Squadrito, 70 F Supp 2d 868 (ND Ill 2000).
Grubbs v Bradley, 552 F Supp 1052 (MD Tenn 1982).
Hendrix v Faulkner, 525 F Supp 435 (ND Ind 1981).
Dawson v Kendrick, 527 F Supp 1252, 1289 (SD W Va 1981).
Feliciano v Barcelo, 497 F Supp 14, 64 (DPR 1979).
Coldsby v Carnes, 365 F Supp 395, 401 (WD Mo 1973).

E. Laundry

Principle: Adequate facilities or services for the processing, handling, storage, and transportation of soiled linen and soiled clothing and of clean linen and clean clothing must be provided.

Public Health Rationale: Clean clothing and bed linens are essential to minimize the spread of communicable diseases, skin diseases such as tinea (ringworm), and parasites such as lice.

Satisfactory Compliance:

1. There must be an adequate supply of linen, which must be handled and stored to minimize contamination from surface contact or airborne deposits. Soiled linen must be collected in such a manner as is necessary to avoid microbial dissemination into the environment. It must be placed into bags or containers at the site of collection. Separate containers that can be washed and sanitized must be used for transporting unconfined or loose clean and soiled linen.

2. The laundry area, when located in the institution, must be planned, equipped, and ventilated to prevent the dissemination of contaminants and must meet the current CDC guidelines. Soiled linen from health service isolation areas must be double bagged and identified. Suitable precautions must be taken in its subsequent processing. Laundry protocol defines chemicals, water temperatures, and cycle requirements. A wash-water temperature of greater than 160°F (for 25 minutes) or washing with a sanitizing agent such as bleach must be used unless other approved temperature and process is specified. Hot-cycle drying further reduces the microbial contamination of laundry and should be used.

3. Correctional and prisoner laundry workers must wash their hands after handling contaminated laundry and must not be permitted to eat, drink, or smoke in the workplace. All staff must be trained in universal precautions. Universal precautions must be practiced in the laundry area.

4. Infection control inspections in non-medical areas must include the laundry areas.

5. Institutions using commercial linen processing must require that the company providing the service maintain the same standards outlined in this publication. Furthermore, the company must ensure that clean linen is protected from contamination during delivery to the premises. Following cleaning, laundry and linen must be free of irritating agents or chemicals.

6. Clothing or bedding in disrepair must be replaced or repaired. Clothing, bedding, mattresses, and pillows must be cleaned and sanitized before being reissued to a new user.

References

Hospital Infections Program home page: www.cdc.gov/ncidod/hip/default.htm

Johnson C. The correctional setting. In: *APIC Curriculum for Infection Control Practice.* St. Louis, MO: Mosby Year Book; 1996.

Legal References

Campbell v McGruder, 580 F Supp 521, 544 (DC Cir 1978).

Dawson v Kendrick, 527 F Supp 1252, 1288-1289 (SD W Va 1981).

Marhnez Rodriguez v Jimenez, 409 F Supp 582, 591 (DPR 1976).

Coldsby v Carnes, 365 F Supp 395, 401-402 (WD Mo 1973).

Jones v Wittenberg, 323 F Supp 93, 96, supplemental opinion at 330 F Supp 707 (ND Oh 1971).

F. Lighting

Principle: Lighting must be provided in living, working, dining, and recreational areas at levels adequate for staff and prisoner safety and for the maintenance of hygiene and good sanitation.

Public Health Rationale: Adequately illuminated living and working areas are beneficial to prisoners' general psychological well-being. Proper lighting also reduces eye strain and glare, and helps prevent headaches. Maintenance of adequate illumination minimizes the risk of accidents and is conducive to the performance of work tasks and recreation activities and is essential for hygiene and sanitation.

Satisfactory Compliance:

1. For various work tasks, illumination of work surfaces must conform to the standards of the American Society of Illuminating Engineers. The following minimum standards must be met:

Area	Minimum Light Intensity (Foot-candles)
Reading and Study Rooms	30
Living Areas	30
Food Preparation Surfaces and Utensil Washing Area	20
Toilets and Washrooms	20
Bulk Food Storage Areas	10
Exit Ways	10
Nighttime Supervision	3 to 5

2. Improvised light shades in cells and dormitories must not be allowed due to danger of fire. Light bulbs, fixtures, and windows must be clean and in good repair to optimize light penetration. Posters, pictures, draperies, clothing, and similar objects must not obstruct light. Wall and ceiling finishes must be selected to minimize glare. Lighting in cells must be individually adjustable. Whenever possible, the prisoner should have control of the lighting levels in his or her cell. Where prisoners are observed for health problems, safety, or risk of suicide, a minimum of 3 to 5 foot-candles of light are required at all times.

3. Prisoner rooms and cells must provide access to natural light.

See standards developed by the American Society of Illuminating Engineers and the American Institute of Architects.

Legal References

Keenan v Hall, 83 F3d 1083 (9th Cir 1995).
Hoptowit v Spellman, 753 F2d 779, 784 (9th Cir 1985).
Shepherd v Ault, 982 F Supp 643 (ND Iowa 1997).
Jones v City & Co. of SF, 976 F Supp 896, 915-916 (ND Ca 1997).
LeMarie v Maass, 745 F Supp 623, 626 (D Or 1990), *vacated on other grounds,* 12 F2d 1444, 1458-1459 (9th Cir 1993).
Grubbs v Bradley, 552 F Supp 1052 (MD Tenn 1982).
Dawson v Kendrick, 527 F Supp 1252, 1288 (SD W Va 1981).
Laaman v Helgemoe, 437 F Supp 269, 310 (DNH 1977).

G.   Plumbing

Principle: The plumbing system must include fixtures, potable water supply, and wastewater disposal components that conform to national plumbing standards (referenced below).

Public Health Rationale: The supply of safe drinking water and the safe disposal of wastewater, including sewage, are critical for the maintenance of health and the control of waterborne, foodborne, and vectorborne diseases.

Satisfactory Compliance:

1. Water, soil, and waste drain lines and fixtures must be constructed of acceptable materials and installed in conformance with nationally recognized codes. Hot and cold water supplies must be adequate in quantity and pressure. All fixtures must be kept clean. Approved backflow prevention devices must be provided in accordance with the appropriate plumbing codes. There must be no cross-connections to nonpotable lines. All plumbing, including fixtures and connections, must be maintained in good working order.

2. Hot water temperatures for all showers and hand washing stations must be regulated by automatic mixing valves. The recommended temperature range for such facilities should be 105°F to 120°F. Hand washing facilities in cells must have combination faucets or mixing valves. Metered faucets, where provided, should provide an uninterrupted water flow of at least 30 seconds. (Instantaneous self-closing faucets are not acceptable.) In lieu of continuous flow sinks, jails and prisons may provide sinks with stoppers that can plug sinks for water collection. Foot-, knee-, or wrist-operated controls must be provided for lavatories in health care units.

3. Facilities must be equipped, in all classification of housing, to allow people with disabilities access to sinks, showers, toilets, and drinking water.

Legal References

Williams v Griffin, 952 F2d 820 (4th Cir 1991).
Tillery v Owens, 907 F2d 418, 423 (3rd Cir 1990).
Hoptowit v Spellman, 753 F2d 779, 783 (9th Cir 1985).
Jones v City & Co. of SF, 976 F Supp 896, 910 (ND Ca 1997).
Grubbs v Bradley, 552 F Supp 1052 (MD Tenn 1982).
Dawson v Kendrick, 527 F Supp 1252, 1287-1288 (SD W Va 1981).
Lightfoot v Walker, 486 F Supp 504 (SD Ill 1980).
Jones v Wittenberg, 323 F Supp 93, 96, *supplemental opinion at* 330 F Supp 707 (ND Oh 1971).

H.   Solid Waste Collection and Handling

Principle: Solid wastes must be collected, stored, and disposed of in a manner that will not create unhealthful conditions, fire hazards, unnecessary odors, or offer food or harborage to insects, rodents, and other vermin. Handling of infectious waste must be consistent with national and local community standards for infection control.

Public Health Rationale: Proper handling of solid waste is necessary to prevent unhealthful conditions, such as contamination of food preparation and storage areas, fire hazards, harborage for vermin, or injuries to handlers. Proper disposal is necessary to prevent air, water, and land pollution. Infectious waste must be handled properly to reduce the spread of disease and infections.

Satisfactory Compliance:

1. All refuse (garbage and rubbish) must be stored in an orderly manner. Refuse contaminated with or containing organic matter must be stored in clean, durable, leak-proof, nonabsorbent containers, and kept tightly covered. All refuse must be removed to a well-drained location that is maintained in a sanitary condition. Collection of refuse must be made as frequently as necessary to minimize fire hazards, odors, or other nuisances. Rubbish must be regularly removed from hallways, cellblocks, corridors, and other common areas and placed in a collection or disposal site. Under no circumstances should rubbish be accumulated in vacant cells within an occupied area. Refuse should be disposed of in a manner acceptable to the regulatory authority.

2. Hazardous wastes that may contain toxic or explosive chemicals or biohazards must be collected, stored, transported, and disposed of separately and in compliance with provisions of the Resource Conservation and Recovery Act, the Toxic Substances Control Act, medical waste regulations, and other state and federal regulations.

Cross Reference

Communicable Diseases, VI.A

Legal Reference

Feliciano v Barcelo, 497 F Supp 14, 64 (DPR 1979).

I.   Vermin Control

Principle: The exterior and interior premises must be maintained free of vermin infestations, harborage, and breeding sites.

Public Health Rationale: Insects, rodents, and other vermin may serve as reservoirs and vectors of disease.

Satisfactory Compliance:

1. Primary emphasis is placed on cleanliness and on elimination of breeding and harborage places. Facilities must be inspected monthly by trained staff to monitor the effectiveness of vermin control programs. Written records of these inspections must be kept for one year. Evidence of infestations such as visual sightings, tracks, excreta, eggs, egg-case shells, larvae, and carcasses must result in pest control measures.

2. Facilities must be maintained to prevent vermin access. All doors and windows must be tight fitting and screened. Cracks and crevices must be sealed. Drains must be covered and cleaned regularly. (Note: Integrated pest management (IPM) is an excellent, comprehensive system of vermin control that could be adopted by jails and prisons and if properly implemented would meet these standards. Information regarding IPM systems can be obtained from USEPA Office of Pesticide Programs.)

3. All chemicals used in the pest treatment program must be kept in their original containers (properly stored and with the original label intact) and must be used in accordance with label safety instructions. Only staff trained to handle and use insecticides, rodenticides, and similar chemicals should handle chemicals. Such individuals must be licensed under the provision set forth in the Federal Insecticide, Fungicide, and Rodenticide Act of 1972. Documentation regarding location, date, and type of treatment, including chemicals used, must be maintained.

Cross Reference

Communicable Diseases, VI.A

Legal References

Williams v Griffin, 952 F2d 820 (4th Cir 1991).
Tillery v Owens, 907 F2d 418, 423 (3rd Cir 1990).
Hoptowit v Spellman, 753 F2d 779, 783 (9th Cir 1985).
Ramos v Lamm, 639 F2d 559, 569 (10th Cir 1980).
Hendrix v Faulkner, 525 F Supp 435 (ND Ind 1981).
Laaman v Helgemoe, 437 F Supp 269 (DNH 1977).
Coldsby v Carnes, 365 F Supp 395, 401-402 (WD Mo 1973).

J.   Wastewater Collection and Disposal

Principle: All sewage and other wastewater must be collected, treated, and disposed of in a manner that will not endanger human health or wildlife or create a nuisance, consistent with local, state, and federal standards.

Public Health Rationale: Improper treatment and disposal of wastewater has been linked to groundwater and surface water pollution and to the transmission of waterborne diseases. In addition, improper handling and disposal of human waste in such a manner as to permit contact by humans, animals, and insects may also result in transmission of disease agents.

Satisfactory Compliance:

1. Sewers must collect all wastewater without overload, overflow, or bypass of the treatment system.
2. The design, operation, and management of onsite treatment systems must meet regulatory requirements of the health or environmental protection agency having jurisdiction.
3. Where onsite treatment consists of a wastewater treatment plant or septic tank and leaching system, the system must be located distant from areas subject to flooding, isolated from drinking water supplies, consistent with federal and state standards, and must be properly supervised by a licensed operator.

Legal References

Williams v Griffin, 952 F2d 820 (4th Cir 1991).
Pritchett v Page, No. 99 C 8174 (ND Ill 2000).
Jones v City & Co. of SF, 976 F Supp 896, 910 (ND Ca 1997).
Nilsson v Coughlin, 670 F Supp 1186 (SD NY 1987).
Anderson v Redman, 429 F Supp 1105, 1112 (D Del 1977).

K.   Water Supply

Principle: A safe and adequate water supply must be provided.

Public Health Rationale: An adequate supply of potable water is necessary for health, personal hygiene, and sanitary purposes, and for fire fighting requirements.

Satisfactory Compliance:

1. The water supply must be of sanitary quality and adequate in quantity to meet the institutional demands, including fire fighting, without significant reduction in water pressure. If the supply is obtained from a municipal source, microbiological and chemical quality should be monitored at the treatment plant and in the water distribution system; however, an employee with environmental orientation must conduct periodic sanitary surveys of the internal water distribution system at least annually to check for and eliminate potential backflow and back siphonage from any plumbing fixture or connection to nonpotable water through cross-connections or other means. Such employees must have demonstrated competency in testing backflow prevention devices and in recognizing cross-connections.

2. For onsite systems, the water quality, quantity, source, treatment, storage, distribution, and pressure must meet the provisions of the Safe Drinking Water Act, including sampling frequency, operator certification, operation, maintenance, monthly reporting on operation, watershed surveillance, cross-connection control, and water system sanitary survey evaluation. The water supply must be under surveillance of the appropriate regulatory authority that regulates the public water supply.

3. Drinking fountains must be of the sanitary angular jet type if single service drinking cups are not provided. There must be readily accessible drinking water fountains in all living areas.

4. Nonpotable piped water (if available) must be carried in a separate, clearly labeled piping system and may not be accessible for drinking.

Legal References

Leenan v Hall, 83 F3d 1083 (9th Cir 1995).
Masonoff v DuBois, 899 F Supp 782 (D Mass 1995).

X.C FACILITIES

A.   Recreational Facilities

Principle: Safe, sanitary, adequate, and suitable indoor and outdoor recreation space, facilities, and programs that have been adapted to the prevailing weather conditions must be provided.

Public Health Rationale: Recreation facilities, coupled with a moderate exercise program and leisure-time activities, are conducive to improved physical and mental health.

Satisfactory Compliance:

1. Outdoor recreation areas must be level and adequately drained. There must be at least 15 square feet of space per prisoner for the maximum number of

prisoners expected to use the space at one time, but not less than 1,500 square feet of unencumbered space. In facilities with a population of less than 100 prisoners, 750 square feet of unencumbered space is adequate.

2. There must be adequate indoor or, in warmer climates, covered recreation space to accommodate all prisoners in inclement weather. Indoor recreation areas must be at least 18 feet high and provide a minimum of 35 square feet per prisoner for the maximum number of prisoners who may use the indoor space at one time. Dayrooms do not qualify as recreational space for the purposes of meeting this standard.

3. All recreation areas must have ready access to showers, toilets, lavatory facilities, and sanitary drinking fountains or single service drinking cups. Where a bathing beach or swimming pool is provided, it must comply with the state health department rules and regulations. All facilities must be safe and must be maintained in a clean and sanitary condition. Policies must define minimum recreational opportunities for the prisoner population. The recreation schedule must be modified when security and safety of the facility is threatened or in cases of inclement weather.

4. Jails and prisons must provide recreation options that allow for large muscle and aerobic exercise for at least one hour per day for every prisoner.

Legal References

Keenan v Hall, 83 F3d 1083 (9th Cir 1995).
Tillery v Owens, 907 F2d 418, 423 (3rd Cir 1990).
Martin v Sargent, 780 F2d 1334, 1338 (8th Cir 1985).
Hoptowit v Ray, 682 F2d 1237 (9th Cir 1982).
Campbell v Calithron, 623 F2d 503 (8th Cir 1980).
Campbell v McGruder, 580 F Supp 521, 544-546 (DC Cir 1978).
Smith v Sullivan, 553 F2d 373 (5th Cir 1977).
Amaker v Goord, 98 Civ 3634 (SD NY 1999).
Hendrix v Faulkner, 525 F Supp 435, 525 (ND Ind 1981).
Heitman v Gabriel, 524 F Supp 622 (WD Mo 1981).
Lightfoot v Walker, 486 F Supp 504 (SD Ill 1980).

B.   Facilities Available to the Public

Principle: Facilities for the public must include adequate waiting room space, toilet facilities, and a sanitary drinking fountain or single-service drinking cups. Facilities for the handicapped must be provided as specified in barrier-free design requirements as specified by the Americans with Disabilities Act.

Public Health Rationale: Adequate toilet facilities and drinking fountains or single-service drinking cups that are conveniently located are necessary for personal health and hygiene and to minimize the spread of disease. Facilities must be barrier-free to encourage visiting by family and friends who require such accommodations.

Satisfactory Compliance:

1. Toilet facilities should be within 100 feet of public areas served and the number of plumbing fixtures provided for each sex is based on the maximum number of visitors accommodated as follows:

Number of Visitors	Number of Toilets	Number of Lavatories
1–15	1	1
16–35	2	2
36–55	3	3
56–80	4	4

Urinals may be substituted for up to one third of the toilets for men. Toilets must be in separate compartments. Construction and appurtenances must meet plumbing code requirements.

2. A sanitary drinking fountain or a single-service drinking cup dispenser must be provided for every 75 persons.

3. At least one toilet, sink, and drinking fountain in each visiting area must be barrier-free.

4. There must be a safe and sanitary area for changing infants.

Legal References

Ramos v Lamm, 639 F2d 559 (10th Cir. 1980) *cert. denied* 450 US 1041 (1981).
Marhnez Rodriguez v Jimenez, 409 F Supp 582, 589 (DPR 1976).

C.   Barber and Beauty Shops in Institutions

Principle: Barber and beauty shops must be designed, operated, and maintained in a sanitary manner consistent with local standards for barber and beauty shops in the community.

Public Health Rationale: Skin diseases and ectoparasites may be transmitted either through direct contact or by objects such as towels, combs, clippers, or razors.

Satisfactory Compliance:

1. Barber and beauty shops must be maintained in a clean and sanitary condition. Combs, clippers, razors, and similar objects must be routinely sanitized between uses. Prisoners with evidence of communicable disease or head lice or those whose face, neck, or scalp is inflamed must not be served. Instead, these prisoners must be referred to the health care clinic for treatment. Employees must have adequate training, be free of communicable disease, wear clean attire, wash hands with soap and running water before attending to each prisoner, use individual sanitary neck-strips and towels, and follow other hygienic practices. Common dusters, brushes, and mugs must not be used. The facilities must comply with local standards for community based barber shops or beauty parlors.

2. Time-release faucets, light, ventilation, and facilities for the physically disabled must comply with requirements listed in other sections of these standards.

Legal Reference

Hendrix v Faulkner, 525 F Supp 435, 489 (ND Ind 1981).

X.D SAFETY

A. Environmental Controls for Injury Prevention

Principle: Facility construction, alteration, and operation must consider safety principles and concepts. Adequate records of all injuries should be required to effectively control future injuries.

Public Health Rationale: Accidents account for a large number of the injuries that require treatment and that may cause temporary or permanent disability to the prisoner and financial cost to the community.

Satisfactory Compliance: The same principles of injury prevention that apply to any institution, plant, workplace, or home must apply to a correctional institution. The following accident prevention guidelines must be met:

1. Design, maintenance, and arrangement of facilities, including the surface finishes and lighting, must minimize hazards of falls, slipping, and tripping. Handrails must be provided on stairs and ramps. Safety glass must be used in doors and walls. Doors used as emergency exits must swing open in the direction of the exit.

2. Protection must be provided against all electrical hazards, including shocks and burns.

3. Design, installation, and maintenance of fuel-burning and heating equipment must minimize exposure to hazardous or undesirable combustible materials and must minimize risk of fire or explosion.

4. Facilities must be provided for the safe and proper storage of drugs, insecticides, flammable liquids, poisons, detergents, and any other substances that could cause injury if not properly stored and used. All such substances must be properly labeled.

5. The environment must be controlled to minimize burns from hot water, steam, uninsulated contacts, unshielded or uninsulated hot pipes, or radiators. Under no circumstances should hot water exceed 120°F in showers and lavatories (110°F is recommended) and steam-mixing valves for such fixtures are expressly prohibited. **NOTE:** Hot water of 135°F can cause third-degree burns in 10 to 15 seconds. Consumer Product Safety Commission recommendations must be met.

6. In colder climates, walkways must be maintained to minimize slipping on snow and ice.

7. In work areas, safety devices must be in place and proper clothing, including proper shoes, must be worn by all prisoners to minimize injuries, cuts, burns, contact with chemicals, and eye injuries.

8. OSHA standards must be met for prisoners, correction officers, staff, and visitors.

9. Records of all accidents and injuries must be kept by medical staff. Records must be reviewed monthly by medical and institutional staff and action must be taken to prevent recurrences.

Cross Reference

Injuries, IX.A

Legal References

Tillery v Owens, 907 F2d 418, 424 (3rd Cir 1990).
Masonoff v DuBois, 899 F Supp 782 (D Mass 1995).

B. Disaster Planning

Principle: Disaster planning must be adequate to assure safety of staff, prisoners, and visitors.

Public Health Rationale: Disasters, whether man-made or naturally occurring, may result in hysteria, injuries, and loss of life.

Satisfactory Compliance:

1. Disaster planning must include written provisions for disasters that result from earthquakes, tornadoes, floods, riots, explosions, and fires. The disaster plan must include specific actions for utility breakdowns such as loss of heat, water, and electricity.

2. A disaster plan must be maintained and available to key officials. Unless security is compromised, prisoners must be moved during disaster drills. Upon arrival in a living unit, a prisoner must be informed as to how to respond during a disaster. Signs showing routes of emergency egress should be posted in all areas of the jail or prison.

3. Disaster drills that involve personnel responsible for maintaining utilities and services must be conducted on an annual basis. The results must be documented and changes must be implemented where indicated. Communications for the purpose of managing disasters must be established with local and state disaster planning officials. Disaster planning activities, including the roles of local or state planners, must be documented.

Legal References

Jones v City & Co. of SF, 976 F Supp 896, 909 (ND Ca 1997).
Ruiz v Estelle, 503 F Supp 1264, 1382 (SD Texas 1980).
Feliciano v Barcelo, 497 F Supp 14, 38 (DPR 1979).

C. Fire Protection and Fire Safety Practices

Principle: Fire protection and fire safety practices must be adequate to protect life and prevent injury.

Public Health Rationale: The security requirements of the prisoner population, the potential for internal disturbances that may result in fire, and the limitations of free movement and exits in correctional facilities require that materials used within the facility be fire safe, that fire control services and early detection devices be readily accessible, and that fire prevention techniques and procedures be strictly followed. Smoke inhalation is a major cause of fire-related deaths.

Satisfactory Compliance: All structures, facilities, and equipment must be constructed and maintained in accordance with applicable fire protection standards. The following specific criteria must be met:

1. All construction and finishes must be fire-resistant. Fabrics and drapes, including privacy curtains, must be certified as fire-resistant and combustible furnishings must be minimized.

2. Areas containing combustibles and potentially flammable vapors must be posted and kept free of open flames. Such areas must be inspected at least monthly to ensure compliance.

3. The use of polyurethane mattresses is prohibited. Mattresses must be constructed of fire-retardant treated cotton, neoprene foam, or equivalent.

4. Flammable liquids must be properly stored.

5. Chutes, shafts, stairs, kitchens, boiler rooms, incinerator rooms, paint and carpenter shops, and similar hazardous rooms must have fire-resistant enclosures.

6. Passageways, doors, and stairs must be of proper width and be marked, kept clear, enclosed, and compartmented as required by applicable fire and building codes. Adequacy is dependent on the number of prisoners and staff, the number of floor levels and the height of the building, fire protection equipment, and other factors. All prisoners and staff must be able to exit safely from the building in case of emergency.

7. Two remote fire exits must be provided; dead-end corridors are prohibited.

8. Automatic sprinklers must be located in chutes, soiled linen areas, trash and storage rooms, and in any areas for the handicapped, disabled, or medically infirm (e.g., the infirmary).

9. Automatic fire suppression systems must be provided in kitchen hoods, shops, and storage rooms and must be inspected and tested by qualified persons at frequencies stated in local or national fire codes. Records of these inspections and the findings must be kept for at least one year.

10. Fire-fighting apparatus, facilities, and alarms must be adequate for the facility and readily available, and their location and use must be known to all staff. Fire hydrants, hoses, and standpipes must be operable. Fire extinguisher number, type, location, condition, and recharge data must meet applicable code requirements set by state and/or local fire safety authorities and the National Fire Protection Association's Life Safety Code.

11. Smoke detection systems must be provided in sleeping areas, in areas of public assembly, and in the boiler room, kitchens, laundry, garage, paint and carpenter shops, and other work areas in the facility. The internal fire alarm system must be connected to the fire department or station. Fire-rated smoke detectors or alarm-activated self-closing fire-rated doors must be installed between smoke compartments. The alarm and detection systems must also shut off the ventilation system when it is likely smoke will be introduced into areas not affected by the fire and/or smoke.

12. A sufficient number of self-contained, positive-pressure breathing apparatuses must be available and located in the facility and meet the requirements of the local or state fire marshal.

13. Correctional officers must maintain visual surveillance of prisoner living areas when doors are not provided with remote-release capability. All prisoner living areas must have exit doors provided with remote-release capability. Smoke dampers, self-closing doors, and egress to fire and smoke compartments must meet the National Fire Protection Association's Life Safety Code requirements.

14. Fire drills should include building evacuation when possible and must be conducted at least twice annually for each shift and the results must be documented. Evacuation plans must be posted at suitable locations.

15. Adequate fire safety training for correctional officers and institution employees must be provided during orientation and in-service training annually thereafter.

16. There must be a manual override for electric cell doors. If keys are required to open cell doors, the keys must be readily available to staff at all times.

D. Institutional Operations

Principle: All prison and jail institutional maintenance and on-premises industries or manufacturing must comply with the applicable federal and state safety standards that are comparable to private sector operations.

Public Health Rationale: Safe, sanitary, and healthful working conditions, processes, and procedures are essential to prevent injury, illness, disability, and death.

Satisfactory Compliance: Canning, dairy, milk and food processing, and ice-making must comply with FDA standards; meat and slaughterhouse operations must comply with USDA standards; hospital operations must comply with Department of Health and Human Services standards; water works, sewage works, and solid waste management operations must comply with federal and state standards; and manufacturing and other work-related operations must comply with current OSHA standards.

Cross Reference

Occupational Health, IX.B

Legal References

Tillery v Owens, 907 F2d 418, 424 (3rd Cir 1990).
Carty v Farrelly, 957 F Supp 727 (DVI 1997).
Jones v City & Co. of SF, 976 F Supp 896, 908 (ND Ca 1997).
Masonoff v DuBois, 899 F Supp 782 (D Mass 1995).
Inmates of Occoquan v Barry, 269 F2d 210 (DC Cir 1988).
Cody v Hillard, 599 F Supp 1025 (SDSD 1984).
Heitman v Gabriel, 524 F Supp 622 (WD Mo 1981).
Grubbs v Bradley, 552 F Supp 1052, 1073 (MD Tenn 1980).
Owens-El v Robinson, 457 F Supp 984 (WD Pa 1978).

E. Noise Control

Principle: Facility design, maintenance, and operations must include consideration of noise and vibration control.

Public Health Rationale: Excessive noise causes irritation, mental and emotional strain, and distraction that may result in increased risk of injury. Noise of sufficient intensity and duration can cause hearing loss, interfere with speech and communication, and contribute to unrest and injuries.

Satisfactory Compliance:
1. Noise levels should not exceed acceptable levels given the level of activity in the institution and time of day. Where available, the services and advice

of a governmental agency with expertise in noise assessment and control must be used to evaluate the significance of apparent or alleged noise problems and advise on corrective actions.

2. Noise levels within prisoner living areas should not exceed 70 decibels in the daytime and 45 decibels at night. Noise levels should be monitored and documented periodically.

3. Noise levels must meet OSHA standards for all workplace environments.

Legal References

Keenan v Hall, 83 F3d 1083 (9th Cir 1995).
Jones v City & Co. of SF, 976 F Supp 896, 908 (ND Ca 1997).
Toussaint v McCarthy, 597 F Supp 1388, 1397, 1410 (ND Ca 1984), *aff'd in part, rev'd in part on other grounds,* 801 F2d 1080, 1110 (9th Cir 1986).
Anderson v Redman, 429 F Supp 1105, 1112 (D Del 1977).

F. Radiation Safety

Principle: Ionizing radiation exposures must be reduced to the lowest achievable level consistent with contemporary national standards for public health and safety.

Public Health Rationale: The control of exposures to ionizing radiation, including medical, dental, industrial process, and other applications, is necessary to minimize the risk of cancer, germ cell damage, and chromosomal aberrations.

Satisfactory Compliance:
1. All radiation equipment must be routinely inspected and tested in accordance with the standards of the presiding health agency.
2. Personnel operating radiation equipment or handling ionizing radiation sources must have documented training and certification in safe operating practices as specified in Public Health Law 97-35 of the Consumer-Patient Radiation Health and Safety Act of 1981. Safety rules must prescribe safe practices and personnel should receive in-service safety training annually. Non-dental or non-medical exposures that occur in worksite environments should be limited to the levels set by OSHA standards.

X.E HYGIENE AND PERSONAL REQUIREMENTS

A. Personal Hygiene

Principle: All practical measures must be taken to control communicable diseases such as ringworm and pediculosis. Prisoners should have adequate grooming supplies and an area in which to groom themselves.

Public Health Rationale: Ringworm of the scalp, body, nails, or feet is communicable and may cause baldness and lesions on various parts of the body, including the hands and feet, and may also lead to secondary infections. Supplies and facilities for personal hygiene and grooming should promote cleanliness and minimize the possibility of infection and illness.

Satisfactory Compliance:
1. Institutions should follow control measures outlined in the current *Control*

of Communicable Diseases Manual, 17th Edition (American Public Health Association, 2000).

2. Clean towels must be issued to each prisoner upon admission to the institution and restocked at least three times per week.

3. Each prisoner must be provided with toothpaste or powder, a toothbrush, soap, and comb, and each should have access to shaving gear.

4. Toilet paper must be provided to all prisoners and all female prisoners must be issued sanitary napkins and/or tampons when they are needed.

5. If prisoners do not have adequate clothing, suitable clothing must be provided. Washable clothing must be laundered at least once a week. Clean clothing and bedding must be provided more frequently when medically indicated. Prisoners must also have three complete changes of clothing weekly. Provision must be made to issue additional clothing essential for prisoners who perform special work assignments such as food service, or medical, farm, or maintenance duties. Appropriate clothing must also be provided for outdoor recreation in cold weather.

6. Facilities must be available in sufficient supply to meet the personal hygiene needs of the prisoner population. Showers must be available and prisoners must be permitted access to the showers daily for at least a 5-minute interval unless limited by written security policies. Prisoners should always be allowed at least two showers each week.

7. Frequent hand washing should be encouraged to prevent the spread of disease.

8. The denial of access to sanitary facilities must not be used as a means of punishment.

Legal References

Mitchell v Maynard, 80 F3d 1433, 1442 (10th Cir 1996).
Keenan v Hall, 83 F3d 1083 (9th Cir 1995).
Martin v Sargent, 780 F2d 1334, 1338 (8th Cir 1985).
Inmates of Allegheny Co. Jail v Wecht, 565 F Supp 1278 (WD Pa 1983).
Dawson v Kendrick, 527 F Supp 1252, 1288-1289 (SD W Va 1981).
Hendrix v Faulkner, 525 F Supp 435, 525 (ND Ind 1981).
Heitman v Gabriel, 524 F Supp 622 (WD Mo 1981).
Grubbs v Bradley, 552 F Supp 1052, 1075 (MD Tenn 1980).
Lightfoot v Walker, 486 F Supp 504 (SD Ill 1980).
Feliciano v Barcelo, 497 F Supp 14, 63 (DPR 1979).
Palmigiano v Garrahy, 443 F Supp 956 (DRI 1977).
Anderson v Redman, 429 F Supp 1105, 1112 (D Del 1977).
Marhnez Rodriguez v Jimenez, 409 F Supp 582, 589 (DPR 1976).
Coldsby v Carnes, 365 F Supp 395, 401 (WD Mo 1973).

B. Bedding

Principle: Bedding must be provided to each prisoner except when the medical staff feels it may represent a safety hazard to the prisoner.

Public Health Rationale: Regularly issued, clean bedding provides for health maintenance and minimizes illness and infection.

Satisfactory Compliance: Each prisoner must be provided a bed, clean mattress, a pillow, a pillow case, a blanket, and a sheet and mattress cover (or two sheets). The sheets, mattress cover, and pillow case must be changed weekly. Blankets must be cleaned weekly if used by multiple prisoners or whenever visibly soiled, or annually if used by one prisoner in a prison. All bedding, including mattresses, must be sanitized between users according to methods approved by the CDC.

In situations in which a prisoner is judged by the medical staff as a suicidal risk, bedding should be withheld temporarily (see Suicide Prevention, V.E) pending a full mental health evaluation (within 12 hours). However, bedding should not be withdrawn or withheld as a matter of punishment.

Legal References

Mitchell v Maynard, 80 F3d 1433, 1442 (10th Cir 1996).
Campbell v McGruder, 416 F Supp 100 (DDC 1975).
Toussaint v Rushen, 553 F Supp 1365 (ND Cal 1983).
Dawson v Kendrick, 527 F Supp 1252, 1288-1289 (SD W Va 1981).
Hendrix v Faulkner, 525 F Supp 435, 525 (ND Ind 1981).
Heitman v Gabriel, 524 F Supp 622 (WD Mo 1981).
Lightfoot v Walker, 486 F Supp 504 (SD Ill 1980).
Palmigiano v Garrahy, 443 F Supp 956 (DRI 1977).
Anderson v Redman, 429 F Supp 1105, 1112 (D Del 1977).
Coldsby v Carnes, 365 F Supp 395, 401 (WD Mo 1973).
Jones v Wittenberg, 323 F Supp 93, 96 (ND Oh 1971).

C.   Toilet and Bathing Facilities

Principle: Toilets, lavatories, and bathing facilities must be adequate and suitable for the population housed in a prison or jail.

Public Health Rationale: Toilets, lavatories, and bathing facilities are essential to the maintenance of health and the prevention of disease.

Satisfactory Compliance: Adequate numbers of properly-connected, well-maintained sanitary facilities must be available. The following fixtures and facilities must be provided:

1. Individual flush toilet or equivalent and lavatory for each cell.
2. If prisoners are housed in dormitories, flush toilets in the ratio of 1 to every 8 prisoners and lavatories in the ratio of 1 to every 8 prisoners.
3. Shower facilities in the ratio of 1 to every 8 prisoners as well as soap and individual towels.
4. Tempered water must not exceed 120°F in the showers and lavatories (temperature should be set at 110°F).
5. Adequate supply of toilet paper.
6. Safety mirror in each lavatory.
7. Sanitary-type drinking fountains for each cell block floor or single-service drinking cups for each cell.
8. Adequate flush toilet and lavatory facilities for assembly, work, school, recreation, food preparation, dining, and similar areas.
9. Service sinks for each cell block.

10. Hot and cold or tempered water for each lavatory in dormitories or other living areas.
11. In men's dormitories, urinals may be substituted for up to one third of the toilets.

D. Space

Principle: Sufficient space that is appropriate to the task or area function must be provided.

Public Health Rationale: Adequate space is necessary to minimize the spread of communicable disease, carry out certain tasks, minimize stress and injury, provide for privacy, and contribute to health maintenance, safety, and general well-being.

Satisfactory Compliance:

1. Single cells or rooms must be available to house prisoners when required by institution policies, or when prisoners may be endangered by other prisoners and request separation. Such areas must have a minimum of 60 square feet of floor space and an 8-foot-high ceiling, except when prisoners are locked in for more than 10 hours a day; then there should be a minimum of 70 square feet of floor space and an 8-foot-high ceiling.
2. The use of double-occupancy cells is strongly discouraged. If used, they must provide a minimum of 120 square feet of floor space and must have at least 8-foot-high ceilings.
3. Use of double-deck bunks in cells or in dormitories is not recommended and must never be used if ceiling height is less than 10 feet. When double bunks are used, guard rails must be provided.
4. Dormitories must provide a minimum of 60 square feet of floor space per prisoner and must have 8-foot-high ceilings except when prisoners are locked in for more than 10 hours a day; then there should be a minimum of 70 square feet of floor space per prisoner and at least an 8-foot-high ceiling. A non-obstructed evacuation route for use in emergencies must be maintained.
5. Double-occupancy beds, or use of a single mattress for two prisoners, is not permitted except where conjugal visits are permitted.
6. Day rooms must be provided contiguous to each dormitory or cell block. At least 35 square feet of unencumbered floor space per prisoner must be provided and ceilings should be at least 8 feet high.

Legal References

Ramos v Lamm, 639 F2d 559, 567-569 (10th Cir 1980).
Cody v Hillard, 599 F Supp 1025 (SDSD 1984).
Toussaint v Rushen, 553 F Supp 1365 (ND Cal 1983).
Hendrix v Faulkner, 525 F Supp 435, 525 (ND Ind 1981).
Feliciano v Barcelo, 497 F Supp 14, 66-68 (DPR 1979).
Laaman v Helgemoe, 437 F Supp 269, 309-310 (DNH 1977).
Anderson v Redman, 429 F Supp 1105, 1112 (D Del 1977).

X.F INSPECTIONS, PERSONNEL, AND SUPERVISION

A.   In-Service Training

Principle: Institutional staff who are responsible for environmental health and sanitation must be trained for the supervisory roles to which they are assigned.

Public Health Rationale: Defects or deficiencies in the physical environment can result in hazardous situations that may result in illness or injury to the prisoners and staff. In addition to environmental risks typical of institutional living, correctional institutions have certain conditions that accentuate these risks or that may present hazards unique to these institutions. Therefore, surveillance must be conducted by adequately trained personnel to identify and minimize these risks.

Satisfactory Compliance:

1. Institutional personnel must receive training that is comparable to that provided for supervisors and employees of community facilities. Training must be planned by and, if possible, provided by the staff of the appropriate government agency (e.g., the health department, environmental protection agency, or occupational health and safety agency) and should be provided in the same manner as training is provided to workers in the community.

2. Institutions must designate a qualified individual and provide adequate staff and support services to conduct environmental surveys and outline corrective measures (staff and support is dependent on the size of the facility). This person(s) must be directly responsible for all environmental sanitation and must ensure that the sanitation of the facility meets all state licensing or registration requirements for public health sanitarians.

B.   Self-Inspection

Principle: Trained, qualified jail or prison staff should conduct frequent environmental surveys. The frequency of such surveys must be dictated by the magnitude of public health hazard and be in compliance with written policies. All areas of the jail or prison must be inspected at least monthly by a public health sanitarian. In addition, there must be formal inspections and consultations provided by state and local regulatory agencies.

Public Health Rationale: Because much of the risk resulting from unsanitary or unsafe environmental conditions is the consequence of human factors (e.g., neglect, carelessness, ignorance, and oversight) it is essential to provide maximum surveillance of critical operations and activities. Self-inspection is especially important to ensure acceptable living and working conditions within institutional environments.

Satisfactory Compliance: There must be written policies and procedures that describe the frequency and content of regular health and safety self-inspections and to ensure compliance with all environmental sanitation provisions detailed in these standards. Deficiencies must be noted and actions must be documented. Copies of written inspection reports and remedial action taken must also be provided to responsible managers as defined by institutional policy and as indicated in the quality improvement program. Time frames for corrective action must be set, met, and monitored and records must be retained onsite for at least 5 years.

C.   Regulatory Agencies

Principle: Public health, fire, occupational safety and health, and other agencies that have similar regulatory responsibilities must be invited to make biennial facility-wide inspections and to file reports to the responsible institution administrator, agency, or board or commission regarding the health environmental engineering and sanitation of the institution.

Public Health Rationale: Environmental health engineering and sanitation inspections and recommendations (when followed) can minimize the incidence of preventable illness and death due to poor hygiene and the environment.

Satisfactory Compliance:

1. A minimum of biennial and preferably annual inspections must be made by agencies that have similar responsibility to the public. The inspections must be carried out without hindrance and reports and recommendations must be made to the responsible institution administrator, agency, and board or commission. The regulatory inspection must cover the areas in the environmental health sections of these standards.

2. Deficiencies must be documented and a specific plan to correct them must be developed and implemented. Time frames for corrective action must be set, met, and monitored.

Cross References

Health Care Facilities, II.E
Communicable Diseases, VI.A

Glossary ─────────────────────────

Administration of medication: the act in which a single dose of a medication is given to a patient.

Correctional authority: an agency, regardless of name, that is ultimately responsible for operating the jail, prison, or youth facility.

Dispensing of medication: the act of placing proper doses of prescribed medication into labeled containers that indicate the name of the patient, the contents of the container, and other necessary information.

Health authority: the government entity, regardless of local name, that is ultimately responsible for the health services provided to incarcerated persons at an institution or system of institutions. In some instances this will be a health services unit within a larger department of corrections. In others, this will be a government health department.

Health care provider: clinical staff including physicians, physician assistants, nurses, and other health care staff who are licensed and trained to provide health care services. Health care providers do not include the non-clinical and administrative staff.

Health care staff: all trained and licensed health care providers and other secretarial or administrative support staff who work in or for the health care program. Custody or security staff who may be assigned to medical areas of a jail or prison are not included in this term.

Hospice: Hospice services provide support and care for persons in the last phases of incurable disease so that the dying may live as fully and comfortably as possible. Hospice recognizes dying as part of the normal process of living and focuses on maintaining the quality of remaining life; it neither hastens nor postpones death. An underlying tenet of hospice is that with appropriate care and a caring community sensitive to their needs, patients and their families may be free to attain a degree of mental and spiritual preparation for death that is satisfactory to them.[1]

Independent licensed health care provider (ILHCP): A physician, physician assistant, nurse practitioner, and any other health care provider who is licensed and certified to diagnose, treat and prescribe medications either autonomously or under physician supervision.

Independent licensed mental health provider (ILMHP): A psychiatrist, physician assistant, or advance practice nurse who is licensed and certified to treat and prescribe medications either autonomously or under physician supervision.

Indigent: a prisoner with no (or minimal) funds in his or her account and no immediate source of funds.

Initial medical screening: Screening done at time of admission to custody by health care staff. This screening is followed within a week's time by a complete medical examination.

Jail or prison: These standards use these terms to refer to the institutions that incarcerate adults or juveniles who are accused of committing delinquent acts and who have been adjudicated delinquent.

Juvenile: a person under the age of twenty-one, or under the age of majority, as defined in a local jurisdiction.

Mid-level provider: An independent licensed provider who is not a physician.

Palliative care: Shares with cure-oriented care the qualities of plan-driven activity, purposeful organization and evaluation, range of treatment options, and care giver-patient engagement and collaborative decision making. The only distinguishing characteristic is the goal of care: palliation has compassionate caring rather than cure as its goal. Because palliation remains on the care continuum after cure is no longer the goal, it may encompass particular comfort measures posing risks to life that might not have been acceptable when cure was still the goal of care.[2]

Prisoner: any person confined in a local, state, or federal jail, prison, or youth facility (for minors alleged to have committed delinquent acts or to have been adjudicated delinquent). (Note: When these standards differentiate between the requirements in jails and prisons, they will make the distinction explicit.)

Receiving screening: see Initial medical screening.

---

1 National Hospice Organization, *Standards of a Hospice Program of Care* (Arlington: National Hospice Organization, 1993).
2 Post LF, Dubler NN, "Palliative Care: A Bioethical Definition, Principles, and Clinical Guidelines," *Bioethics Forum.* 1997;13(3):17-24.

Index ———————————————————

Other Titles of Interest from APHA

Control of Communicable Diseases Manual *(17th Edition)*
Edited by James Chin, MD, MPH
ISBN 0-87553-182-2 • 640 pages • hardcover
ISBN 0-87553-242-X • 640 pages • softcover

Collaborative Research: University and Community Partnership
Edited by Myrtis Sullivan, MD, MPH, and James G. Kelly, PhD
ISBN 0-87553-179-2 • 260 pages • softcover

Communicating Public Health Information Effectively:
A Guide for Practitioners
Edited by David E. Nelson, MD, MPH; Ross C. Brownson, PhD;
Patrick L. Remington, MD, MPH; and Claudia Parvanta, PhD
ISBN 0-87553-027-3 • 240 pages • softcover

Confronting Violence *(Second Edition)*
By George A. Gellert, MD
ISBN 0-87553-001-X • 384 pages • softcover

Public Health Management of Disasters: The Practice Guide
By Linda Landesman, DrPH, MPH
ISBN 0-87553-025-7 • 288 pages • softcover

Caring for Our Children:
National Health and Safety Performance Standards
for Out-Of-Home Child Care *(Second Edition)*
ISBN 0-97156-820-0 • 440 pages • softcover

For more information on APHA books or to order, go to: www.apha.org/media